Complete Ketogenic Diet Guide

Complete Ketogenic Diet Guide For Beginners (With 30 Day Meal Plan and 50+ Recipes)

Introduction

Here is some shocking statistics; according to a study published in the *New England Journal of Medicine,* 54 out of every 100,000 deaths in 2015 were related to being overweight/obese. The study also claimed that obesity caused 4 million deaths in 2015 alone. Shocking huh!

So is there any hope for you as an overweight person or are you just inline waiting to suffer the deadly fate of being overweight?

Well, you will be happy to know there is hope for you so keep reading. You can actually escape the dangers of being overweight and that is by you losing weight.

I know you know the dangers of being overweight and perhaps have tried many things to shed some weight but if you haven't tried the Ketogenic diet yet, this is perhaps the reason why you are still struggling with weight loss!

I say this because the Ketogenic diet works. It works, unlike many other approaches that require daredevil level of willpower to pull off successfully for the long term. And if you simply search for Ketogenic diet or Keto diet on your favorite social media site, you will see scores of stories of real people who are making it with the Ketogenic diet. This alone should fuel your enthusiasm to want to get started immediately.

But you won't lose weight magically just because you have started following the Ketogenic diet. To succeed in your *journey to sustainable weight loss*, you MUST understand the Ketogenic diet inside out so that you know why you have to make different dietary choices. This will ensure that you are knowledgeable on what makes you gain weight and what you must do to lose weight. This knowledge alone will be enlightening, as you can use it to your benefit even if you are on a weight loss plateau.

And if you are wondering what is this I am taking about, this book will introduce you to the inner workings of the Ketogenic diet so that you know what to do and why you should do what you do. After reading this book and taking action, you can bet that weight loss will never seem like an impossible feat for you.

In this book, you will get to learn the basics of the keto diet, benefits of a keto diet and how to get started with the diet. You will also be provided with a 30 day meal plan backed by over 50 recipes to get you started with the Ketogenic diet without getting bored.

Let's get started.

Thanks again for purchasing this book. I hope you enjoy it!

Table of Contents

Before we get to the hows of the Ketogenic diet, let's deal with the whats. We'll start by understanding what the diet is all about.

Basics Of A Keto Diet

As a beginner, you must be wondering what this super diet called a keto diet is and how exactly is it able to help you lose weight without you having to skip a meal. Well, this chapter is going to answer you all those questions; so pay attention as we start.

What Is A Ketogenic Diet?

The Ketogenic diet is basically a way of eating which entails eating food that is high in fat, low in carbohydrate and moderate in proteins.

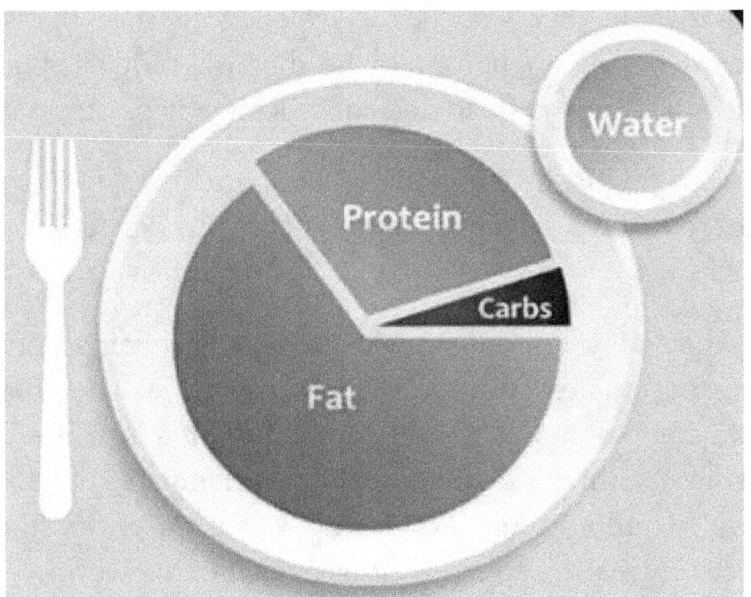

The behind eating this way is to get your body into a metabolic state known as ketosis, a state where your body shifts from relying primarily on glucose for energy to relying primarily on ketones (or ketone bodies) for energy. Since ketones are obtained from the breakdown of fats, this means that the diet is very effective for weight loss (I'll explain how in a bit). Other than that, it reduces the risk of developing such diseases like heart disease, stroke, diabetes, epilepsy and Alzheimer's, as you will come to see later on in this book.

The question you might be having right now is; how is the keto diet able to do all that? For you to understand that, you will first need to learn where the diet came from.

Here is a brief history of the Ketogenic diet.

A Journey Down The Memory Lane

The Ketogenic diet was first developed in the 1920's. But unlike what you might think, the diet was not designed for weight loss. It was instead designed as an epilepsy treatment.

Now you might be wondering how the diet came to be considered as an epilepsy treatment in the first place. Well, here is how.

Thousands of years ago, ancient Greek physicians believed that fasting was essential to a healthy lifestyle. They believed that fasting was so powerful that one could use it to treat almost everything, including health problems like epilepsy. So for over two thousand years, fasting was used as the standard practice for treating epilepsy across much of the world.

In 1911, the first modern study of the role of fasting in epilepsy took place in France. The researchers discovered that periods of fasting combined with low-calorie diet reduced seizures and the effects of epilepsy. Also an American osteopathic physician called Hugh Conklin experimented with fasting around that time by prescribing it to his epileptic patients. The results were amazing, as he got a 50 percent success rate- which went to show that fasting really worked.

But as amazing as fasting was in treating epilepsy, it had one problem. It wasn't reliable. This is because fasting could only be done on a temporary basis. This disadvantage made the doctors to try and find another epilepsy treatment that is reliable and can last for long periods of time.

Dr. Wilder at the Mayo Clinic then came up with the perfect solution. The doctor conducted a research and discovered that epilepsy patients experienced fewer seizures when their blood sugar was low. This discovery encouraged Dr. Wilder to create a diet that is low in blood sugar. That's how he came up with a high fat, low carbohydrate and moderate protein diet by the name of Ketogenic diet.

The keto diet was able to treat epilepsy without the patient having to fast or starve, as it only reduced the intake of carbohydrates. After a few years of using the keto diet as an epilepsy treatment, the diet was abandoned for the newly introduced anti-seizure medication. The keto diet is still effective for treatment of drug resistant epilepsy.

Today, the keto diet is famously used as a way of losing weight. How? We will discuss that next.

How Does The Ketogenic Diet Work?

The time has come for you to get the answer to the question that has been lingering in your mind from the time you heard about the keto diet; 'how does a keto diet work?'

Here is how.

The power behind the Ketogenic diet's ability to help you lose weight and have better health comes from one simple action that the diet initiates in your body once you start following it. This simple action is how the keto diet changes your metabolism from burning carbohydrates for energy to burning fats for energy.

What does that have to do with weight loss and a better health?

Let me break it down for you.

- ***Burning carbohydrate for energy***

Most of the food we eat follows the food pyramid recommended by the USDA some few decades ago. The pyramid puts carbohydrates at the bottom of the pyramid and fats at the top of the pyramid, which essentially means that carbohydrates form the bulk of the foods we eat, as shown below:

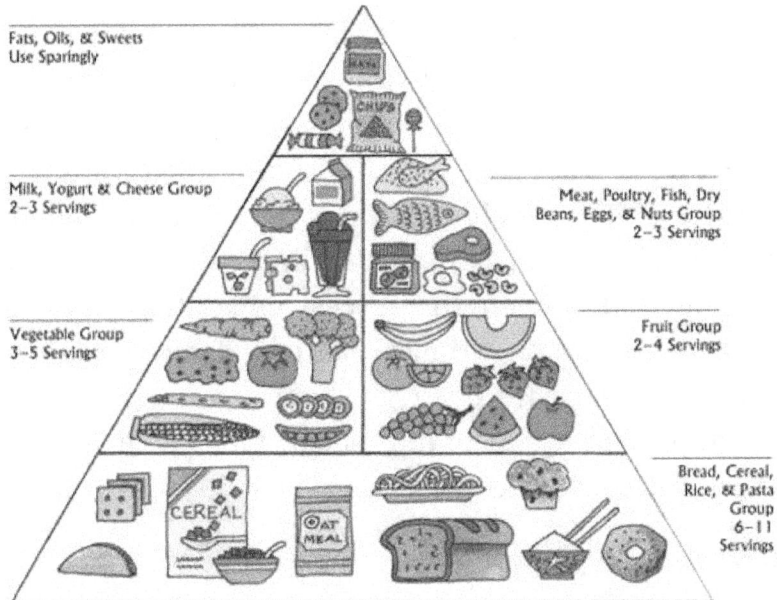

Fats, Oils, & Sweets
Use Sparingly

Milk, Yogurt & Cheese Group
2–3 Servings

Meat, Poultry, Fish, Dry
Beans, Eggs, & Nuts Group
2–3 Servings

Vegetable Group
3–5 Servings

Fruit Group
2–4 Servings

Bread, Cereal,
Rice, & Pasta
Group
6–11
Servings

What many of us don't know is that when you consume a diet that is high in carbohydrate, two things normally happen.

- One, your body takes the just consumed carbohydrates and converts it into glucose which is the easiest molecule that your body can convert to use as energy (glucose is your body's primary source of energy, as it gets chosen over any other energy source in your body).

- Secondly, your body produces insulin for the sole purpose of it moving the glucose from your bloodstream into your cells where it can be used as energy.

There is more that goes unnoticed though:

Since your body gets its energy from glucose (which is mostly in huge amounts owing to the fact that we eat lots of high carb food 3-6 times a day), it doesn't need any other source of energy. In fact, many are the times when glucose is in excess, something that prompts the body to convert dietary glucose

15

into glycogen to be stored in the liver and muscle cells. But since glycogen stores tend to be quite limited, the excess glucose is converted into fatty acids and glycerol, which is stored in fat stores around the body in the form of triglycerides. What this simple explanation means is that with a high carb diet, your body is essentially in what we refer to as a fat storing mode. It store this excess fat so that it can use it when starved from its primary source of energy; glucose. Unfortunately, since we don't give ourselves enough breaks from food, we end up being in this constant fat storing mode that ultimately causes weight gain.

- ***Burning fats for energy***

As you now know, the Ketogenic diet is a low carb, high fat and moderate protein diet. So when you start following a Ketogenic diet, what normally happens is your intake of carbohydrate is kept at a low. In other words, it inverts the USDA food pyramid I mentioned earlier, something that literally 'inverts/reverses' the effects of a high carb diet.

How exactly does it do that?

Well, when you limit your carb intake greatly, you starve the body of its primary source of energy, something that initiates the process that the body has always been preparing for through its energy storage processes. More specifically, the body starts by metabolizing glycogen with the help of glucagon hormone (the process takes place in the liver). And with support from the human growth hormone, cortisol and catecholamines (norepinephrine to be more specific), the body starts releasing fatty acids for use as energy in different body parts. But since fatty acids cannot be used by every cell in the body, the body is also forced to transport some of the fatty acids to the liver where they are broken down in a series of metabolic processes known as ketosis to produce 3 ketone bodies. Ketosis is a normal process that your body activates when your energy intake is low for the purpose of helping you to survive. The three ketones that are formed when fatty acids are converted are:

- Acetone.

- Beta-hydroxybutyric acid (BHB)

- Acetoacetate (AcAc)

Many of your body cells (including the brain cells) can use BHB for energy, as it is water soluble, something that makes it very much like glucose in that it can cross the blood brain barrier. The more ketones the body cells use for energy, the more fat you are burning and ultimately, the more weight you stand to gain. Keep in mind that you are also taking lots of dietary fats. The reason for taking lots of dietary fats is to fill you up fast, make you to stay full for longer and accustom the body cells to using fatty acids and ketones for energy so that when the deficit created by dietary fats kicks in (because you are unlikely to eat too much of fats to the point of meeting your body's energy requirements- unless you are gluttonous), you begin burning stored body fat immediately, as opposed to starting with glycogen. Moderate intake of protein also helps you to get filled fast and to stay full for longer. Make sure to keep your protein intake moderate, as any excess may end up making you to get out of ketosis, as excess protein may be metabolized to glucose in a process known as gluconeogenesis. This essentially means a Ketogenic diet makes your body a fat burning machine, as it relies primarily on fats (both dietary and stored body fat – though you want to get your body to burn as much of the stored boy fat as possible).

Ketosis helps you get rid of excessive fats in your body, which not only reduce your weight in an immense way but also betters your health by protecting you from various diseases as you will see later on.

To attain ketosis, you know that your intake of fats should be high, intake of carbs low and intake of proteins moderate. But what exactly does high, low and moderate translate to in calorie terms? In simpler terms, in what ratios should you take carbs, fats and proteins? This gives rise to several types/approaches/schools of thought regarding the ratios:

Types of Ketogenic diet

As you have seen above, the end goal of a keto diet is to drive you body into a metabolic state of ketosis. Is suggested earlier, there are different ways you can consume a meal high in fats, low in carbs and moderate in protein to reach ketosis. These different ways are what make the different types of keto diet.

Basically there are four types of Ketogenic diets namely:

- ## *Standard Ketogenic diet*

In this type of keto diet, you are made to plan all your meals around fat foods like fatty fish and meats, ghee, butter and avocados. The macronutrient ratio in the standard keto diet is: *75% fat, 15-20% protein and 5-10% carbs.*

- ## *High protein keto diet*

This type of keto diet mainly focuses on increasing your intake of proteins to a substantial amount that does not exceed the intake of fat. The macronutrient ratio in the high protein keto diet is: **60-65%fat, 30% protein and 5-10%** carbs.

- ## *Cyclical keto diet*

This type of a keto diet usually allows you to cycle in and out of ketosis. In short, it lets you follow a keto diet for 5 days and take a break from keto for 2 days in a week. The macronutrient ratio in the cyclical keto diet is:

On keto days: 75% fat, 15-20% protein and 5-10% carbs

On off days: 25% fat, 25% and 50% carbs.

- ## *Targeted keto diet*

This type of keto diet allows you to eat a little more carbohydrate. It is popular among athletes. The macronutrient ratio in the targeted keto diet is: **65-70% fat, 20% protein and 10-15% carbs.**

All the four types of the keto diet are good to use although the most effective one for many people is the standard Ketogenic keto diet.

But does 'many people' suggest that everyone is invited to follow the keto diet? Well, unfortunately, like many things in life, the Ketogenic diet is not for everyone.

Let's discuss more about that next:

Is The Ketogenic Diet For Everyone?

Now that we have established a keto diet is a good tool for weight loss, does it mean that anyone can try it? The answer is no. As unique and as helpful as the keto diet is, it is sadly not safe for everyone.

So who isn't supposed to try the Ketogenic diet? Below is a list of people who should never attempt to reach ketosis or follow a keto diet.

1. *Pregnant or nursing women*

If you are pregnant or a woman who is nursing, you should never try a keto diet because you are at a stage where your body needs to consume more fiber and protein and the keto diet doesn't support that. Why? This is because an increase in protein and fiber usually limits the benefits of a keto diet.

2. *Nutrient deficient or underweight people*

If you are a person who is underweight, the keto diet is not for you. Why? This is because as an underweight person, it's dangerous for you to lose weight and that's exactly what a keto diet will make you do.

3. *A child*

As a child, the keto diet is not for you because the sources of carbohydrates that the keto diet restricts are the same nutrients that you need to grow as a child. Good examples of these carbohydrates include whole grains, dairy and fruits, which all have essential minerals and vitamins.

4. A person with adrenal fatigue

A diet that is moderate in the amount of carb might be helpful for you as a person with adrenal fatigue but one very low in carb such as the keto diet usually worsens the adrenal fatigue. This is because adrenal fatigue is best remedied by a balanced diet, which is hard to have when you are limiting your carbohydrates intake to very low levels.

Now that you have a good understanding of what the Ketogenic diet really is, it's time for you to learn the benefits of a keto diet. Check them out in the next chapter.

What Other Benefits Can You Get From Keto Diet Besides Weight Loss?

I believe the explanation of how the Ketogenic diet works helped you to understand just how it helps with weight loss. That's why I won't talk about that as a benefit (because you already know that). Instead, this chapter focuses on the many other great things that the Ketogenic diet can do for you besides bringing about weight loss. Let's begin.

1. It lowers high blood pressure

In case you don't know, high blood pressure is a very dangerous condition to have, as it predisposes you to life threatening conditions like heart attacks, stroke and heart failures.

But how does it do that?

When you develop high blood pressure, what normally happens is your arteries, the blood vessels that move blood away from your heart to the rest of the body, are hardened due to stress. The hardening then leads to your artery walls thickening, which results to a decrease of blood flow to your heart and an increase of blood pressure. That combination is what normally results to the just mentioned cardiovascular diseases.

The keto diet lowers high blood pressure in your body by dealing with two main culprits of high blood pressure i.e. sugar and salt.

Let me break it down for you.

Sodium and potassium are essential minerals in your body. The two work hand in hand to balance the blood volume and fluid in your body. The thing is; when you eat food that is high in sodium and low in potassium (this is common in the typical American diet), an imbalance automatically occurs. The imbalance then makes your kidney- which is supposed to help you excrete extra fluids- to start holding on to more water. What this does is that it puts pressure on your arteries and increases your blood pressure.

When you follow a keto diet, your blood sugar is usually lowered because you limit your carbohydrate intake. When you lower the sugar in your body, you also lower the salt in your body. How? Blood sugar usually stimulates insulin, which is the substance that promotes the idea of kidney reabsorbing more sodium that leads to high blood pressure. That is how the keto diet eliminates sugar and salt, which results into high blood pressure in your body.

2. It increases your energy levels

The other benefit that you stand to gain once you start following a keto diet is increased energy levels.

As you now know, carbs are converted into glucose, which is absorbed into your cells - through the help of insulin to give you an energy boost. That said, the process of absorbing glucose into your cells doesn't always go as planned.

A lot of times, you get insulin resistance, which is a condition where your cells fail to detect insulin (yes, the cells detect insulin through their insulin detectors – this detection is key in the absorption of glucose into cells). The thing is; when your cells have a problem with insulin detection, this essentially means that the glucose doesn't get to be absorbed into your cells as it should. When this happens, your body releases more insulin into your body in order to get the job done. That results into an insulin spike that creates a rollercoaster of high and low energy levels. The rollercoaster usually leaves you feeling sluggish and hungry and this happens even when you don't have insulin resistance. In short, the energy you get when following a high carb diet is very inconsistent.

When it comes to a keto diet, things are a little bit different. In this case, your body is fuelled by dietary and stored body fat instead of glucose. The good news about that is that fat, unlike glucose, is a constant energy source that never runs out. When following a keto diet, you get to tap into your fat stores at any time your body needs energy. This means with keto diet, you won't get to experience highs and lows in energy levels. You will instead get a consistent level of energy that will keep you on a high always.

3. Fights type 2 diabetes

If you are suffering from type 2 diabetes, you will be happy to know that the Ketogenic diet has the ability to fight the condition. If you didn't know, type 2 diabetes is a chronic condition that occurs when your body doesn't have sufficient production of natural insulin. The condition usually causes high blood sugar in your body.

The Ketogenic diet reverses your type 2 diabetes by doing what all diabetes patients need; control in their blood glucose.

Let me explain:

The high blood glucose level that occurs when you have type 2 diabetes is usually caused by a high intake of carbohydrates. What the keto diet does is that it reduces your carbohydrate intake, which automatically reduces the level of glucose in your blood stream. That is what solves your type 2 diabetes problem.

A study published on Nutr Metab (Lond) in 2008 tried to look at the connection between the keto diet and type 2 diabetes. In the study, 49 diabetes patients were made to follow a low carb diet. At the end of the experiment, the study discovered that low carb diets lead to a great reduction of blood glucose. In fact, the reduction in the experiment was so great that the patients decided to stop their prescribed diabetes medication. That's how good the keto diet is in combating type 2 diabetes.

4. Increases mental clarity

The other benefit of a Ketogenic diet is its ability to increase your mental clarity.

How? Let me break it down for you.

Contrary to popular belief, your brain normally doesn't function that well when your body is using carbs for energy. The reason why this is so is because your body goes through highs and lows in blood sugar levels throughout the day. These highs and lows normally interfere with your energy levels, which automatically affect your brain's focus; and it becomes very hard for you to stay focused for long periods.

The keto diet rectifies your lack of focus and increases your mental clarity by providing your body with a consistent energy supply i.e. fats. When your body uses fats for energy, it enables you to focus for long periods of time.

Obviously, these are not all the benefits that the Ketogenic diet can bring besides weight loss. Others include:

- Helping in the fight against cancer

- Reduction in triglyceride levels

- Improvement of healthy cholesterol (HDL) levels and reduction of unhealthy cholesterol (LDL)

- Fighting against metabolic syndrome

- Improving the health of women with PCOS

- Fighting acne

- Fighting epilepsy

- Protection against degenerative brain diseases like Alzheimer's

- And many others!

Now that you have seen just how good the keto diet is, the question in your mind right now might be; how can I get started? As promised, this book is going to show you how you can get started with the keto diet. But before it does that, we will learn about the 3 macronutrients and their place in Keto diet. Let's get to that in the next chapter.

Keto And Macronutrients

In the beginning of this book, you learned that a Ketogenic diet is a high fat, low carb and moderate protein diet. But as you can tell, that information is too vague to help you as it is.

Let me explain:

If you were today put on a table that had four plates; one containing carbohydrates, the second one containing proteins, the third one containing fats and you were told to use the forth plate, which is empty to serve yourself a keto meal, would you be able to pull it off? The answer is probably not. Why? This is because you don't know how high, low or moderate your fat, carbohydrate and proteins need to be for your meal to acquire the right of being called a keto diet meal.

This chapter is going to help you solve that headache by teaching you about keto and macronutrients.

What Are Macronutrients?

Macronutrients are the nutrients that your body needs in large amounts. Your body usually uses them to produce energy that sustains the wide range of metabolic processes that occur in your body.

There are three types of macronutrients.

- Proteins

- Fat

- Carbohydrates

These three macronutrients are important because their combination in your meals determine whether you will reach the metabolic state of ketosis or not. But what ratio of each are you supposed to take to reach ketosis?

As you are probably aware (we already discussed this earlier when talking about the different types of keto), the best macronutrient intake ratio of the three nutrients for you should be 75**% fat, 20% protein and 5% carbs.** This is the best ratio because it limits your carbohydrate intake to a very small percentage and that makes it easier for your body to switch from using glucose for energy to using fats for energy, which is what you need as a person who is looking to lose weight.

Knowing these percentage ratios is good but they mean nothing in real life, as they are not enough to help you serve yourself a keto meal if you were presented with foods from all the three macronutrients. To eliminate the problem, we will break down the keto ratio of the three macronutrients into a unit that can enable you to make your own keto plate.

How To Calculate Macros While On A Keto Diet

While there are many ways to calculate your macros while on the keto diet, what I have found most convenient is using a macronutrient calculator. This method is efficient because it takes your physique, goals, age and needs into account when calculating your daily keto macros.

With this method, you can know how many grams of each of the three macronutrients you will need to take. So where can you find the calculators? Well, here are some links to good keto calculators that you can use:

- https://calculo.io/keto-calculator

- https://perfectketo.com/keto-macro-calculator/

- https://keto-calculator.ankerl.com/

That said, you can also count your calories manually. Here is how:

✓ Counting your carbs

As a person who wants to lose weight, your daily intake of net carbs should never exceed 30 grams. In fact, for you to lose weight efficiently, you will need to keep your net carb intake at 20 grams.

So, how do you determine your net carb when you are presented with food?

Here is the formula:

Net carb= total carbs − fiber.

So for instance, if you buy food whose nutritional information label states that the total carb is 20 grams and the fiber is 10 gram, it means its net carb is 20 minus 10, which are equal to 10 grams. This means you can eat the food. It also means your allowance for carbs for the rest of the day is 10grams if you don't want to end up kicking yourself out of ketosis.

✓ Counting your protein

Your daily intake of protein usually depends on whether you are looking to build muscles or not. For building muscles, you will need around 1.5- 2.5 grams of protein for every kilogram of your muscle mass. You will need less if you are not interested in building muscles, which can approximately be 0.7-1 gram of protein per pound of muscle mass.

So how can you calculate your daily intake of proteins?

Let's assume you weigh 140 pounds with a 20% body fat percentage.

Step 1: Calculate your body fat by multiplying your weight with your fat percentage.

140 pounds X 0.20(20%) = 28 pounds of body fat

Step 2: Calculate your lean muscle mass percentage by subtracting your body fat percentage from 100.

100 − 20= 80% of muscle mass

Step 3: Calculate the decimal for your lean muscle mass by dividing your muscle mass with 100.

80/100=0.80

Step 4: Calculate total lean mass weight by multiplying the decimal with your total weight.

140 pounds X 0.8= 112 total lean mass

Step 5: Calculate your daily protein intake by multiplying your muscle mass by the grams of protein.

112 pounds X 0.7-1= 78-112 grams of protein per day.

✓ Counting your fat

To calculate your daily fat intake, you will first need to know what calories you need to consume in a day. For you to maintain your current weight as a man, you should consume roughly 2500 calories and if you are a woman, your calorie intake should be roughly 2000 calories. This means that to lose weight, your total calorie intake should be a lot less. But for the purposes of this example, we will use the amount of calories you need to maintain your current weight. Your fat intake should be lower than the figure we get from this example:

Step 1: Calculate the amount of calories that you require for both your carb and protein intake. Using the example above, your protein intake is 78 grams per day and your carb intake is 20 grams per day.

Step 2: Calculate the daily intake of fats.

Since 1 gram of protein and carbohydrate contains 4 calories, it means that the calories from proteins are; 78 X 4= 312 calories. And the calories from carbs are 20 X 4= 80 calories.

The total calories are 312 + 80= 392 calories.

Assuming you are a woman, the calories that you will need in a day are 2000-392= 1608 calories.

Now, 1 gram of fat produces about 9 calories so to get your daily intake, you will divide 1608 by 9 which is 178 grams of fat per day.

Assuming you want to lower your daily calorie totals to 1500 calories (this will be roughly how much you take while on the keto diet since fats and ketones create a satiating effect and keep off hunger and cravings), the new figures will be as follows:

1500-392=1108

1108/9=123.11

So if you weigh 140 pounds and want to lose weight, you should aim to consume about 123grams of fat, 20 grams of carb and 78 grams of protein.

That is how you calculate the three macronutrients and know, which quantity to place on your food in order to reach ketosis.

That said, ketosis is not only triggered by a high intake of fat, low intake of carbs and a moderate intake of proteins. There are other factors that can also help you reach ketosis faster or intensify your fat burning process, which is what you need to lose weight faster. Let's check them out.

How To Reach Ketosis

Here are factors that help you reach ketosis faster apart from you limiting your carb intake, increasing your fat intake and moderating your protein intake.

- ✓ *Fasting-* One of the ways that you can use to reach ketosis or accelerate the intensity at which your body is burning fats is by fasting. Fasting is simply you staying for long hours (anywhere from 14-23 hours is a good place to start) without eating. For example, you can decide not to be eating your breakfast. This will help you get enough fasted hours to get your body to the fasted state where it burns mostly fat.

- ✓ *Stop snacking-* Your body stays in ketosis and burns more weight when there are no insulin spikes. For you to make sure there are no insulin spikes, you will need to stop snacking as that kicks you out of ketosis. Not snacking helps you get and stay in ketosis.

- ✓ *Exercising-* It is known that one of the activities that can help you reach ketosis faster is exercising. Physical activity increases your body's energy demands, which in turn helps you to burn dietary glucose and any stored glycogen to get you into ketosis. And if you exercise when already in ketosis, you burn more fat.

- ✓ *Drinking water-* This may surprise you but drinking a lot of water helps you reach ketosis faster. How? Water is usually amazing when it comes to controlling your hunger pangs. When you drink a lot of water, your desire to snack or even eat normally disappears. This means your carb intake is likely to be low and subsequently, you will get into ketosis a lot faster and stay there. You should aim to drink a gallon of water every day.

✓ *Sleeping enough-* Sleeping for like 8 hours in a day can help you stay in ketosis. How? When you don't get enough sleep, you get stressed and your body releases stress hormones that raise your blood sugar level. This slowly interferes with ketosis. So the opposite, which is having enough sleep, helps you stay in ketosis.

How Do You Know You're In Ketosis?

Here are some of the signs that will tell you that you are in ketosis:

✓ *Dry mouth and thirst-* The first signs of you reaching ketosis is a dry mouth and an increase in thirst. The metabolic state of ketosis makes your body to release a lot of water. That's where the thirst and the dry mouth come from. You should drink a lot of water to avoid being dehydrated.

✓ *Bad breath-* When your body reaches ketosis, it excretes a ketone body called Acetone. This ketone body usually gives you an unpleasant smell in your breath. That's another sign of you reaching ketosis.

✓ *An increase in urination-* As you now know, your body loses a lot of water when in ketosis. So another sign that you will get when you reach ketosis is the feeling of visiting the bathroom regularly.

✓ *Reduced hunger-* When you are in ketosis, your body receives a constant supply of energy from fat, which makes you feel less hungry. So another sign that will tell you that you have reached ketosis is a reduction in hunger.

If you want to be more specific and scientific, you can measure your ketone levels using:

✓ Urine strips: You will be provided with a chart to interpret the results. However, it is not very accurate, as it is often affected by how much water you drink among other factors

✓ Blood ketone meter: You should aim to get a blood ketone meter reading of between 0.5 and 3 mml/L, as this signifies optimal ketosis

At this point, you now know what you need to know before starting the Ketogenic diet. So the next topic is how to get started on a keto diet.

How To Get Started

This chapter is going to take you through a step by step method of how you can get started on a Ketogenic diet. Let's jump straight into it.

Step By Step Method Of How To Get Started In Keto

Step 1: Learn What To Eat And What Not To Eat

To start a Ketogenic diet, you will first need to know what the diet allows you to eat and what it prohibits you to eat. Below are two lists that will educate you on what to eat and what to not eat.

What To Eat When On A Ketogenic Diet

Here are foods you can enjoy on a keto diet.

✓ **Meat, eggs and fish-** almost all fresh meat and fish is good for a keto diet. This includes tuna, salmon, pork, lamb, chicken and beef. The other keto acceptable food that you can enjoy are, eggs, organic meat and wild caught fish.

✓ **Oils and fats-** you are allowed to consume butter, avocado oil, olive oil, bacon fat and coconut oil.

✓ **Dairy**- you can enjoy any full-fat dairy like unsweetened yogurt, cheeses, butter, heavy whipping cream and sour cream.

✓ **Vegetables**- you are required to eat a lot of non-starchy vegetables like zucchini, Brussels sprouts, garlic, tomatoes, cauliflower, peppers, spinach, kale onions, lettuce, cucumber, broccoli, mushrooms and asparagus.

✓ **Fruits**- you are allowed to eat fruits like raspberries, blueberries, and strawberries.

✓ **Seeds and nuts**- you can eat macadamias, walnuts, almonds, pecans, flaxseeds and chia seeds.

✓ **General products**- some of the general foods that you should take include, unsweetened tea, coffee, lots of water, chicken/bone/beef broth, sweeteners like erythritol and stevia and condiments like sriracha, pesto, mustard and mayonnaise.

What Not To Eat

✓ **Vegetable and seed oil**- do not use vegetable and seed oil like grape seed, corn, soybean, safflower and sunflower oil. Also avoid trans fats like margarine.

✓ **Legumes**- avoid lentils, peas, beans and any other form of legume. Also avoid tubers like yams and potatoes.

✓ **Sugary food**- stop consuming products that have refined sugar like candy bars, pastries, milk chocolate, fountain drinks, desserts and fruit juices.

✓ **Starches and grains**- you should not consume wraps, croissants, rolls, bagels, flour, quinoa, oats, corn, potatoes, rice, bread, pasta and cereals.

Step 2: Sanctify Your Kitchen, House And Office

Now that you know what you can and cannot eat, the next step for you is to go inside your kitchen, bedrooms and even your office and remove any type of food that is not allowed in the keto diet. You can place them on a bag to throw away later or to donate to a friend.

This step is important because it enables you to have a fresh start and at the same time, it helps you get rid of unhealthy foods, which can tempt you when they are within your reach or when they are in your face.

If you are not living alone and the other person needs to use unhealthy food, you can sit down with them and come up with a place where he/she can keep his/her foods so that they don't distract/tempt you.

Step 3: Go Shopping

Now that you have thrown out your unhealthy foods, it's time for you to go out and shop for healthy foods that are keto acceptable.

But before you do that, you will need to first sit down with yourself and write down a shopping list.

Here is what to do:

- Make a list of every food that you will need in order to go keto.

- You will then need to walk around your house and take note of the food stuffs that you have and are keto accepted. Cross those foods off your shopping list to remain with a final shopping list.

- Pick your bags and head on to your favorite grocery store.

A lot of people say that keto acceptable foods are expensive. I beg to differ. While it might be a bit more expensive, there are ways that you can use to make them less expensive.

Which ways are these?

✓ One of the things that you can do is to buy food in bulk. When foods are bought in a bulk, they usually come with a discount, which can save you money.

✓ The second thing you can do is to look for stores that have deals on food products. This can save you a lot of money.

Step 4: Create A 30 Day Keto Weight Loss Meal Plan

For you to successfully lose weight when following a keto diet, you must create a keto weight loss meal plan. The reason why this is important is because you are likely not to order food from your favorite restaurant or eat something you are not supposed to eat if you have a meal plan that tells you what you are supposed to eat. When you know what you are supposed to eat and perhaps prepare it beforehand, your chances of eating foods that are not allowed in the keto diet will be low. This will undoubtedly increase your chances of staying in ketosis for longer and losing a lot of weight.

To get you started, this book has a 30 day meal plan, which will be followed by delicious recipes that you can prepare within the 30 day period. You can stretch the meal plan for as long as you want; provided you don't get bored! By the time the 30 days are over (assuming you follow the meal plan strictly), you can bet that you will have lost a significant amount of weight and in the process known your favorite meals so that you can repeat the whole process with your preferred foods.

30 Day Meal Plan

I have broken down the 30 day meal plan into weeks to help you shop with ease for the different foods that you will be cooking every week (assuming you do weekly shopping).

Week 1

Days	Breakfast	Lunch	Dinner
1	Low cab oat meal	Keto chicken salad	Keto chicken with herb
2	Keto Spiced Chai Latte	Salmon filled avocados	Beef bourguignon
3	Bulletproof coffee egg latte	Beef bourguignon leftovers	Mustard lime chicken
4	Keto sausage and eggs	Keto meatballs	Low carb broccoli salad
5	Bacon and eggs	Vegan walnut chili	Cashew chicken fry

6	Keto coffee with cream	Asian cabbage salad	Keto meatballs leftovers
7	Keto chia pudding	Keto spinach Mozzarella stuffed burgers	Keto chicken with herb leftovers

Week 2

8	Keto pancakes	Cashew chicken fry leftovers	Vegan walnut chili leftovers
9	Keto blackberry cheesecake smoothie	Mustard lime chicken leftovers	Keto chicken with herb leftovers
10	Keto egg butter	Deviled eggs	Halloumi cheese with mushrooms
11	Low carb oat meal	Keto no-noodle soup	Pork belly and stir fry kimchi
12	Keto coffee with cream	Asian cabbage salad	Keto meatballs on zucchini noodles. Topped with cream sauce.
13	Sugar free keto blueberry muffins	Keto shrimp and bacon chowder	Keto spinach Mozzarella stuffed burgers
14	Keto sausage and eggs	Zucchini noodles with avocado sauce	Sausage with cilantro lime cauliflower rice

Week 3

15	Keto egg butter	Pizza cups	Cashew chicken fry
16	Keto sausage and eggs	Keto meatballs	Beef bourguignon
17	Keto coffee with cream	Turkey sausage frittata	Low carb broccoli salad
18	Bulletproof coffee egg latte	Keto walnut chili	Creamy cauliflower mashed potatoes
19	Keto pancakes with berries	Zucchini noodles with avocado sauce	Keto chicken with herb
20	Keto blackberry cheesecake smoothie	Salmon filled avocados	Pork belly and stir fry kimchi
21	Bacon and eggs	Keto shrimp and bacon chowder	Halloumi cheese with mushrooms

Week 4

22	Keto blackberry cheesecake smoothie	Keto chicken salad	Low carb broccoli salad
23	Keto spiced chai latte	Vegan walnut chili	Mustard lime chicken
24	Keto egg butter	Keto meatballs	Tomato feta soup
25	Keto pancakes	Asian cabbage salad	Cauliflower rice with cheesy steak roll ups
26	Keto sausage and eggs	Keto spinach Mozzarella stuffed burgers	Pork belly and stir fry kimchi
27	Low carb oat meal	Beef bourguignon	Keto meatballs
28	Keto spiced chai latte with deviled eggs	Goat cheese salad with balsamico butter	Turkey sausage frittata
29	Bulletproof coffee egg latte	Keto shrimp and bacon chowder	Tomato feta soup
30	Sugar free keto	Cashew chicken	Sausage with cilantro lime

	blueberry muffins	fry		cauliflower rice

The above meal plan would be very hard to follow if it wasn't backed by the specific meals mentioned (just imagine how hectic it would be for you to find 'Keto Asian beef salad' directions. Which ingredients would you use? How would you ensure it is keto friendly, as a beginner? To eliminate the hassle of having to find these foods by yourself, the next chapter is dedicated to recipes for the different foods mentioned in the 30 day meal plan and more. Move to the next chapter to get started with the recipes.

Keto Cookbook

Keto Breakfast Recipes

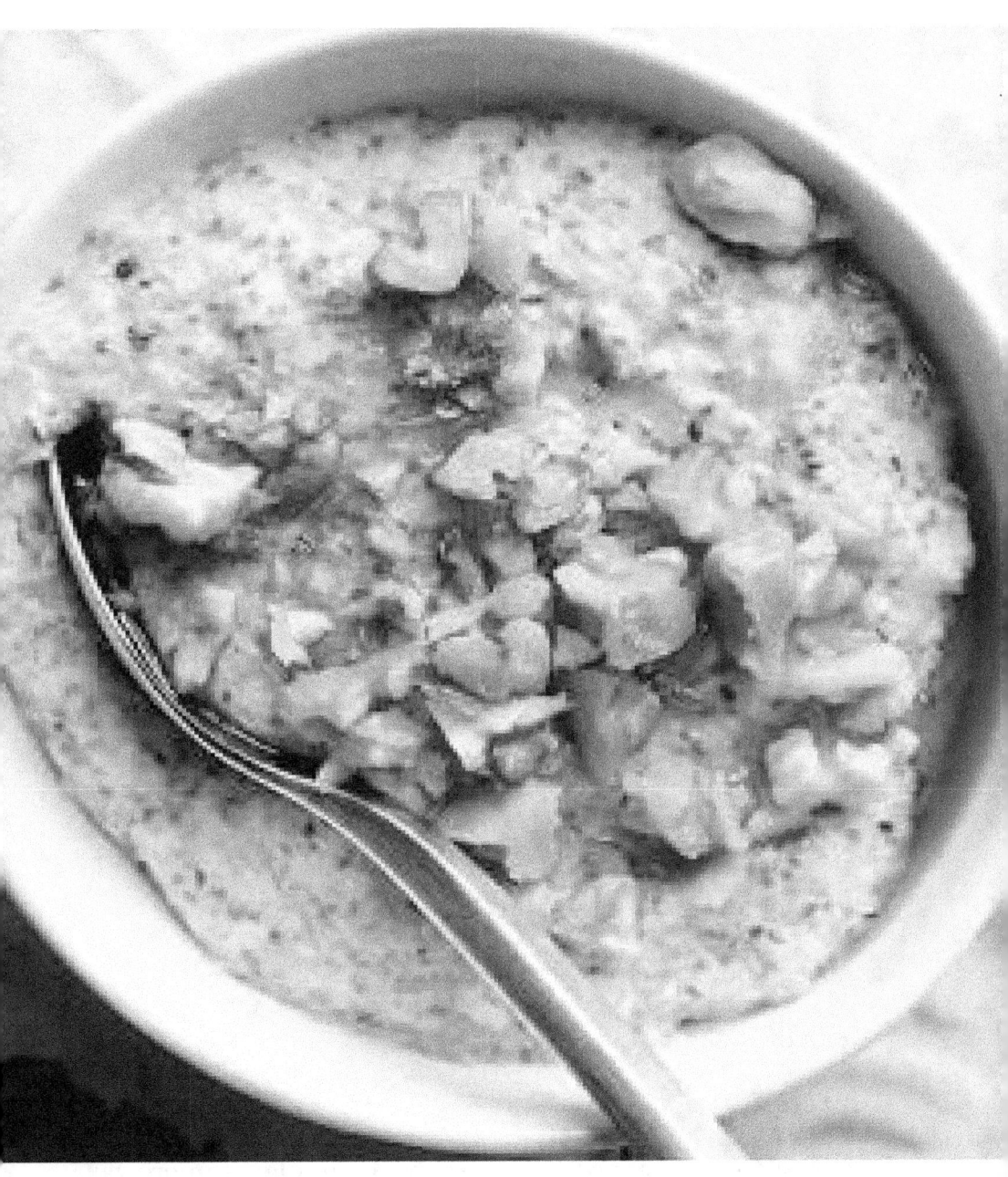

Low Cab Oat Meal

Serves 1

Prep time: 1 minutes, Cook time: 4 minutes, Total time: 5 minutes

Nutritional Information Per Serving: Calories: 453, Proteins: 18g, Carbohydrates: 15g, Fats: 36g

Ingredients

½ teaspoon of pure vanilla extract

A pinch of salt

¼ teaspoon of erythritol blend/granulated stevia or any sweetener of your liking.

1 tablespoon of chia seeds

1 tablespoon of golden flaxseed meal

2 tablespoons of unsweetened shredded coconut

2 tablespoons of almond flour

2 tablespoons of hemp hearts

½ cup of water

Directions

Start with the microwave method: In a large microwave safe cereal bowl, add in all the above ingredients except vanilla. Microwave the combination on high until it thickens.

This should take you about 2 minutes. Stir in the vanilla and serve warm.

Start with the stovetop method: Add all the ingredients except the vanilla into a small saucepan over low heat. Let the mixture cook until it thickens as you stir constantly. This will take you about 3 to 5 minutes.

Stir in the vanilla and serve warm.

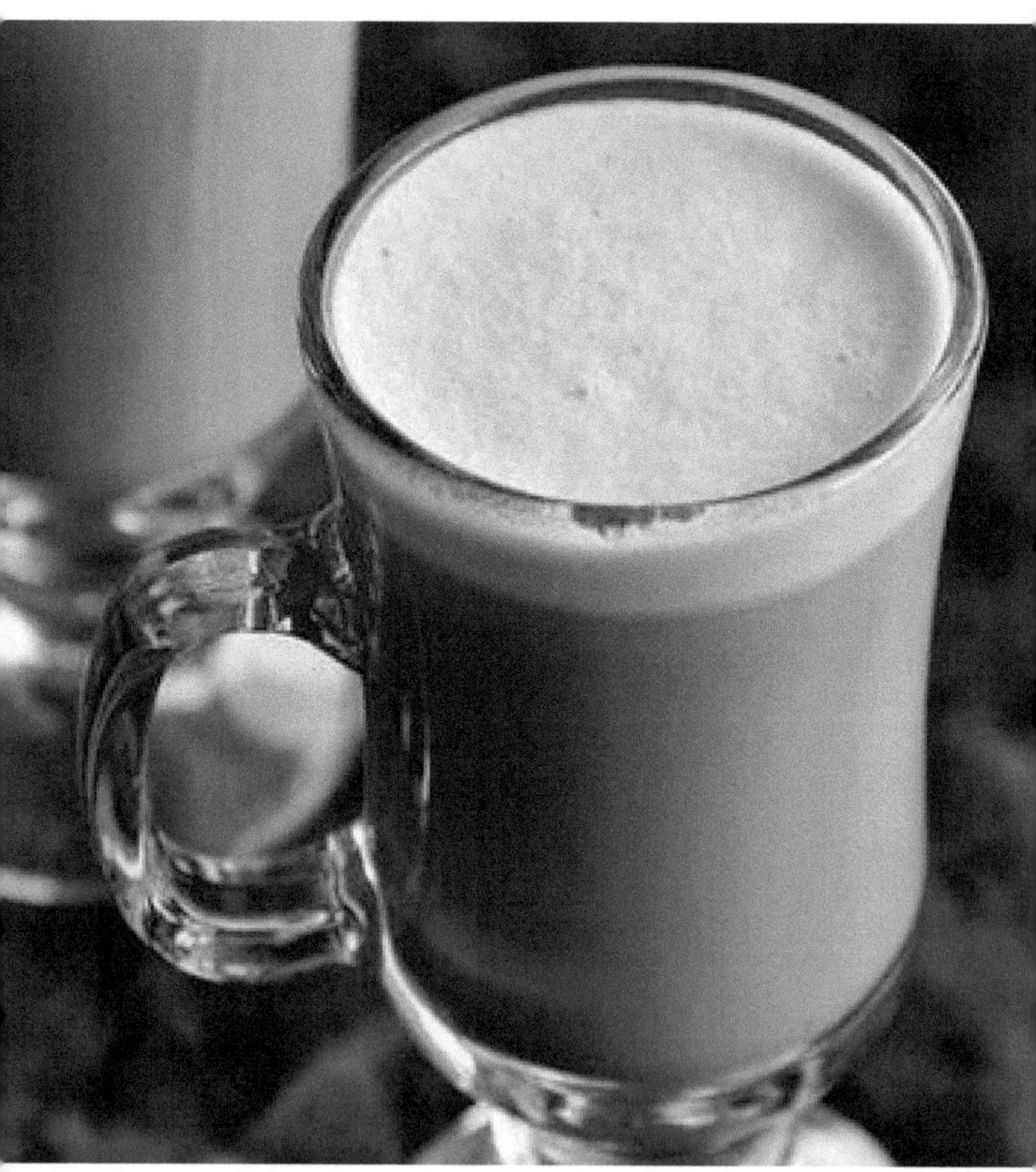

Keto Coffee With Cream

Serves 1

Prep time: 10 minutes, Total time: 10 minutes

Nutritional Information Per Serving: *Calories: 206, Proteins: 2g, Carbohydrates: 2g, Fats: 22g*

Ingredients

4 tablespoons of heavy whipping cream

¾ cup of coffee brewed to your liking

Directions

Start by making your coffee the way you like it.

In a small sauce pan, pour the cream and heat it gently. Stir consistently until it becomes frothy.

Pour the warm cream in a large cup and add in the coffee you made. Stir.

Serve immediately as it is or with a piece of cheese or a handful of nuts.

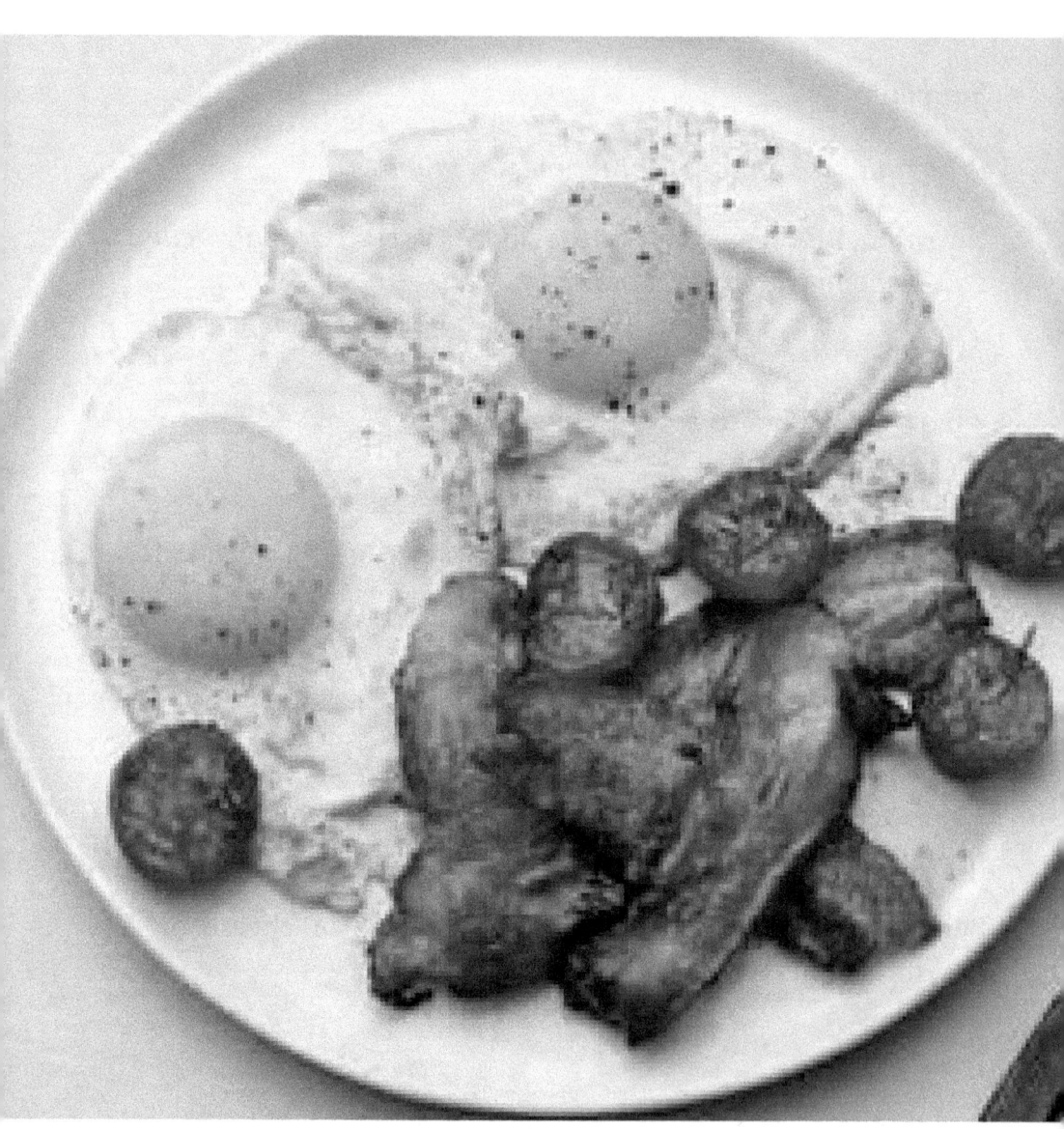

Bacon And Eggs

Serves 4

Prep time: 4 minutes, Cook time: 16 minutes, Total time: 20 minutes

Nutritional Information Per Serving: *Calories: 272, Proteins: 15g, Carbohydrates: 1g, Fats: 22g*

Ingredients

Fresh parsley (optional)

Cherry tomatoes (optional)

5 ounces of sliced bacon

8 eggs

Directions

Start by frying the bacon

Place your bacon in a pan over medium high heat. Fry the bacon until crispy then transfer the bacon on a plate and set aside. The rendered fat should be left in the pan.

Fry your eggs using the same pan

Place the pan over medium heat and crack your eggs open into the bacon grease. If you prefer, you can crack your eggs into a cup and then carefully pour into the pan.

Cook the eggs in your preferred style. If you choose to cook the eggs easy, you can flip the eggs over after a couple of minutes and cook the other side for one minute. If you choose to do a sunny side up, you should leave the eggs to fry on one side and cover your pan so that the top side can cook.

As you fry the eggs, cut the cherry tomatoes into half. Toss them in the eggs and let them fry up together. Garnish with salt and pepper to taste. Transfer to the plate that has the bacon and serve.

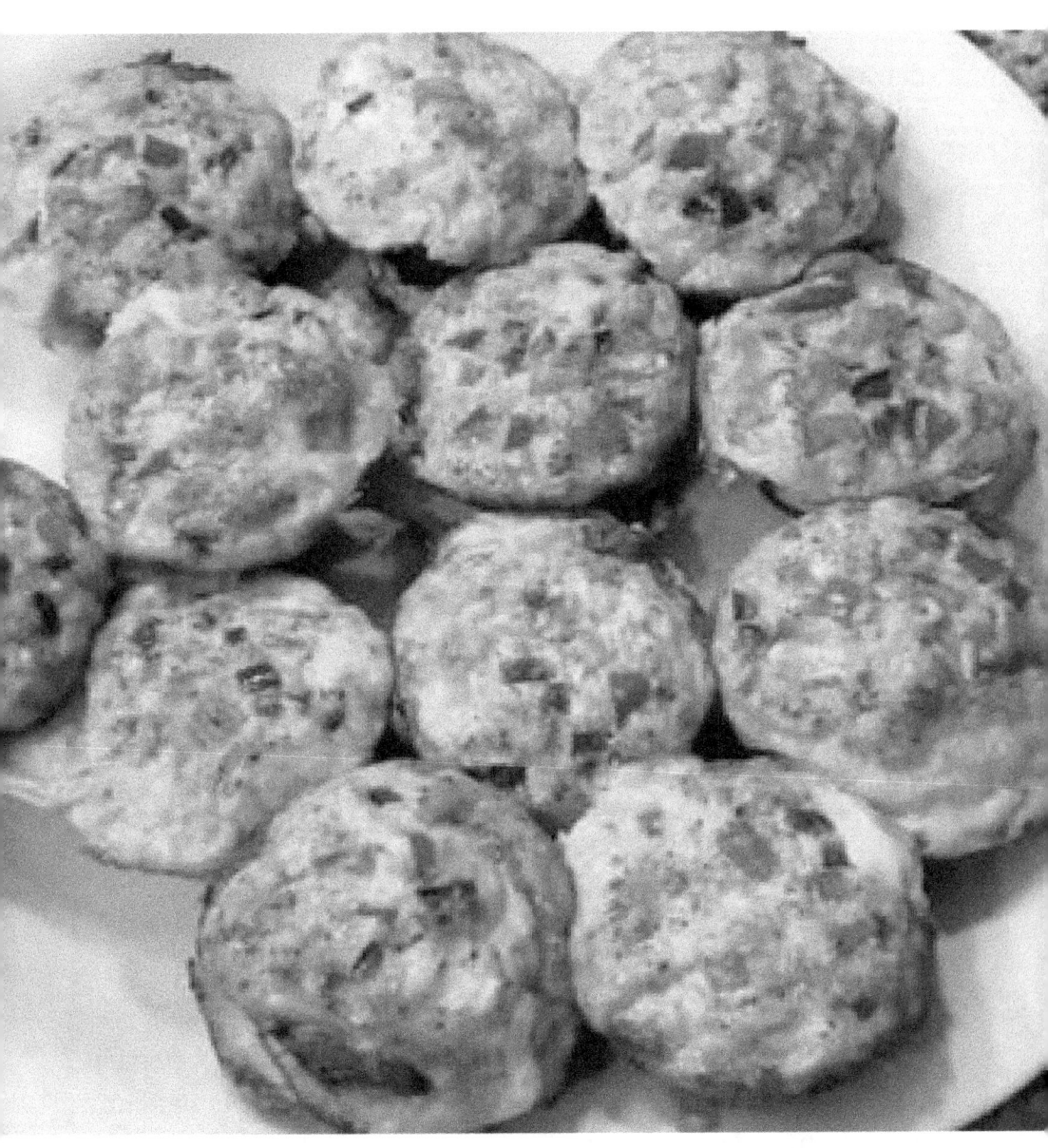

Keto Sausage And Eggs

Serves 4

Prep time: 10 minutes, Cook time: 30 minutes, Total time: 40 minutes

Nutritional Information Per Serving: *Calories: 502, Proteins: 33g, Carbohydrates: 2g, Fats: 39g*

Ingredients

6 eggs

¼ teaspoon of dried parsley

¼ teaspoon of paprika

¼ teaspoon of onion powder

¼ teaspoon of garlic powder

Pepper to taste

Salt to taste

1 lb. of ground sausage, turkey, pork or chicken (455 grams)

Directions

Use a medium sized bowl to combine a mix of dried parsley, paprika, onion powder, garlic powder, salt, pepper and sausage until well combined.

Grease your muffin tin and then start forming shells with the sausage combination that you have just made. The sausage shells must have a room in the middle to accommodate the eggs.

In another bowl, mix eggs with salt and pepper. Pour the mixture in the middle of every cup. Top the cup with toppings of your choice, spinach, tomatoes and shredded cheese.

Place the muffin tin in an oven preheated to 180 degrees Celsius then let the mixture bake for 30 minutes.

Serve and enjoy.

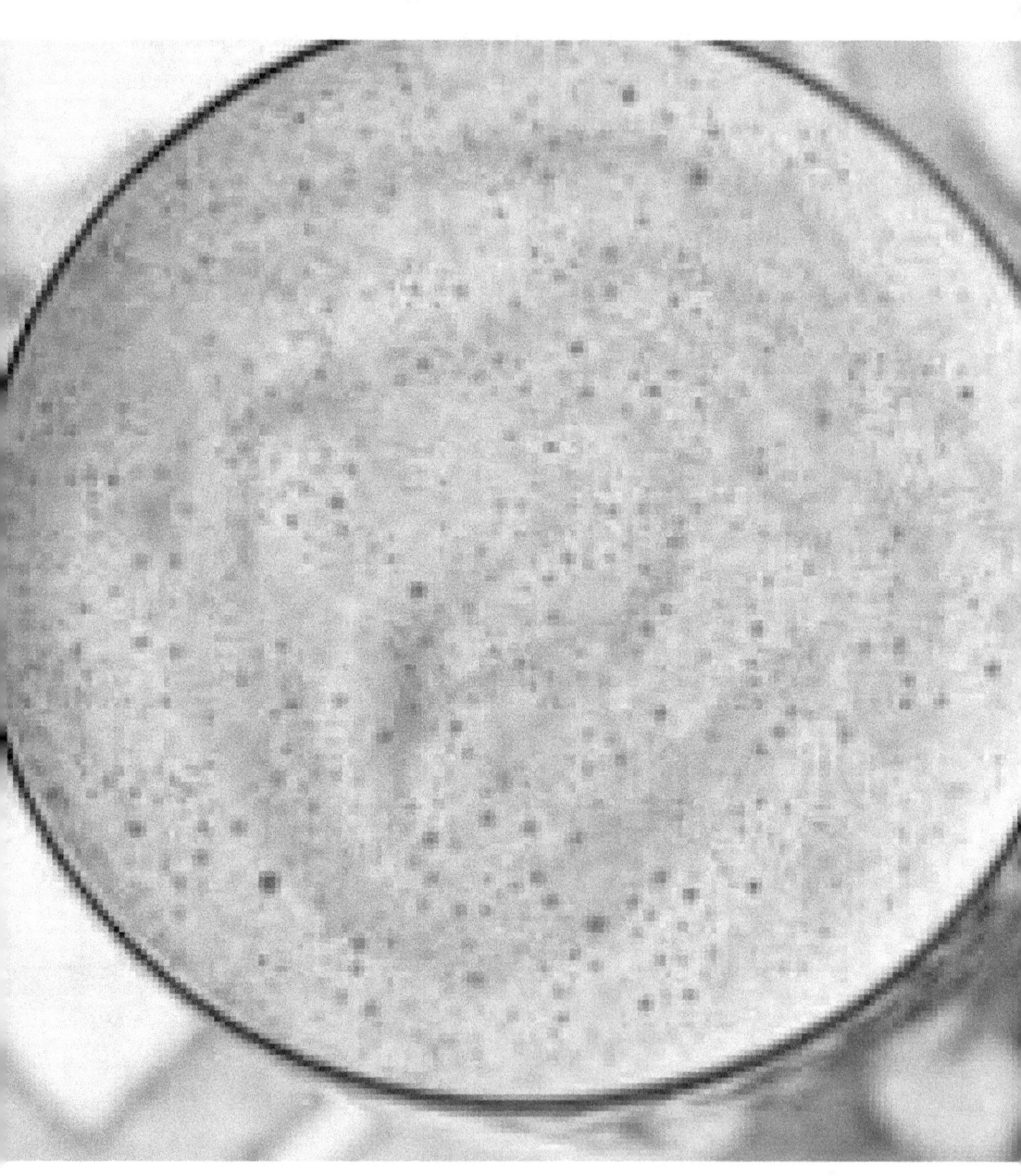

Keto Spiced Chai Latte

Serves 2

Prep time: 7 minutes, Cook time: 3 minutes, Total time: 10 minutes

Nutritional Information Per Serving: *Calories: 105, Proteins: 5.5g, Carbohydrates: 4g, Fats: 8g*

Ingredients

10 ounce of hot water

1 scoop of vanilla collagen protein powder

2 tablespoons of grass-fed ghee or butter

Keto friendly sweetener of your choice to taste

2 pinches of cardamom

½ teaspoon of ginger

¼ to ½ teaspoon of clove

1 teaspoon of nutmeg

½ teaspoon of turmeric

1 teaspoon of cinnamon

1 tablespoon of gelatin (should be bloomed in 2 tablespoons of water)

Optional Add Ins: pinch of cayenne pepper, ½ tablespoon of cacao powder, 1 tablespoon of coconut cream, ½ teaspoon of Ashwagandha, ginseng or other adaptogenic herb of your liking, 1 tablespoon of Brain Octane oil and green or black tea

Directions

Use a small saucepan to gather all the ingredients. Heat the mixture on low heat until the gelatin dissolves.

Pour the mixture into a blender and pulse until frothy. Taste the mixture and adjust the spices and sweeteners.

Pour the mixture into two small cups.

Serve and enjoy.

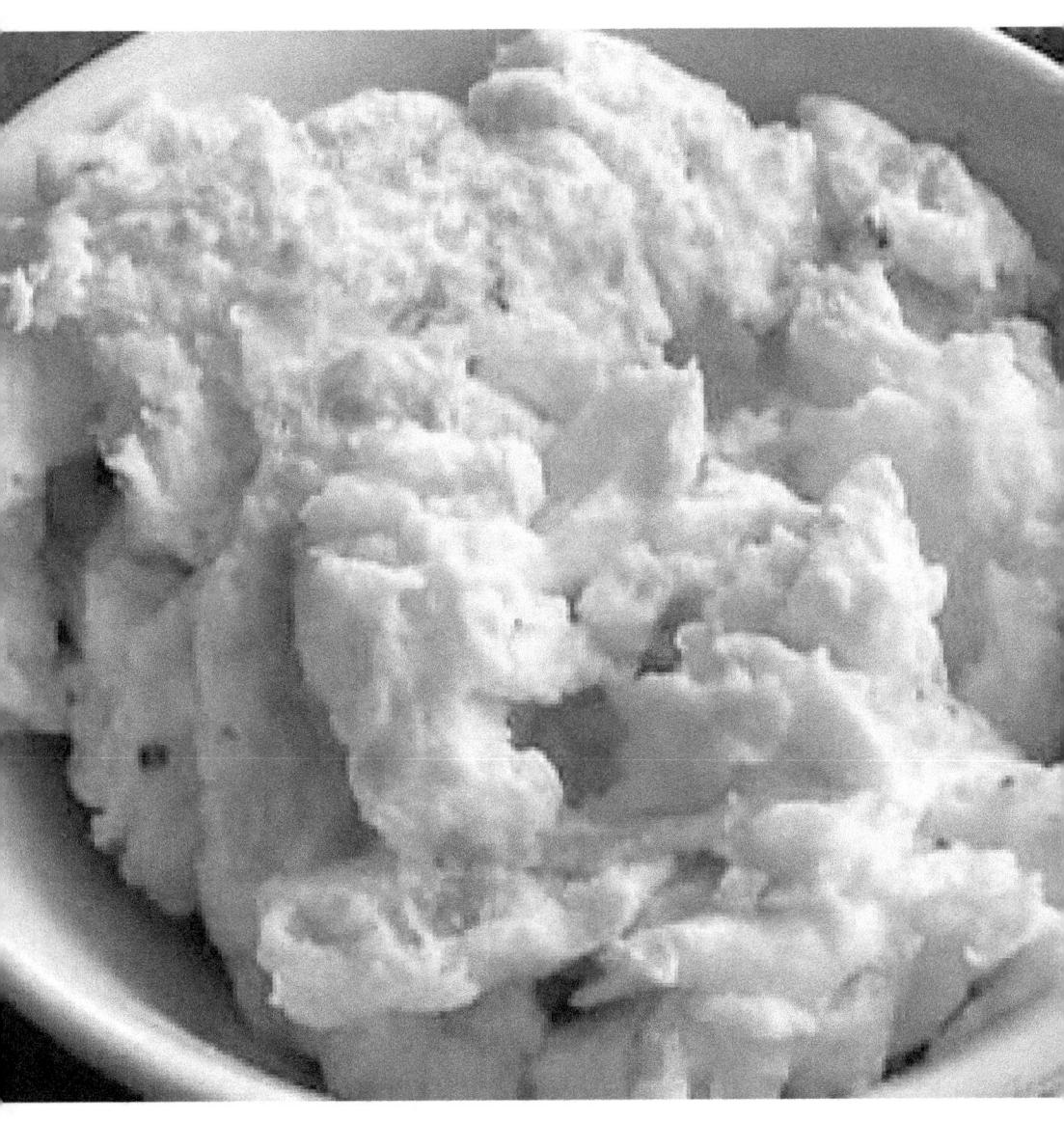

Keto Egg Butter

Serves 2

Prep time: 5 minutes, Cook time: 8minutes, Total time: 13 minutes

Nutritional Information Per Serving: *Calories: 664, Proteins: 12g, Carbohydrates: 1g, Fats: 69g*

Ingredients

¼ teaspoon of ground black pepper

½ teaspoon of sea salt

5 1/3 ounce of butter

4 eggs

Directions

Start by gently placing the four eggs in a pot. Pour in cold water to cover the eggs. Bring to boil without you covering the pot with a lid.

Let the eggs simmer for 8 minutes. Remove the eggs and cool them down in cold water.

Peel the eggs and chop them finely. Stir in salt, pepper and butter. Add any flavoring of your choice (this is optional).

Serve and enjoy.

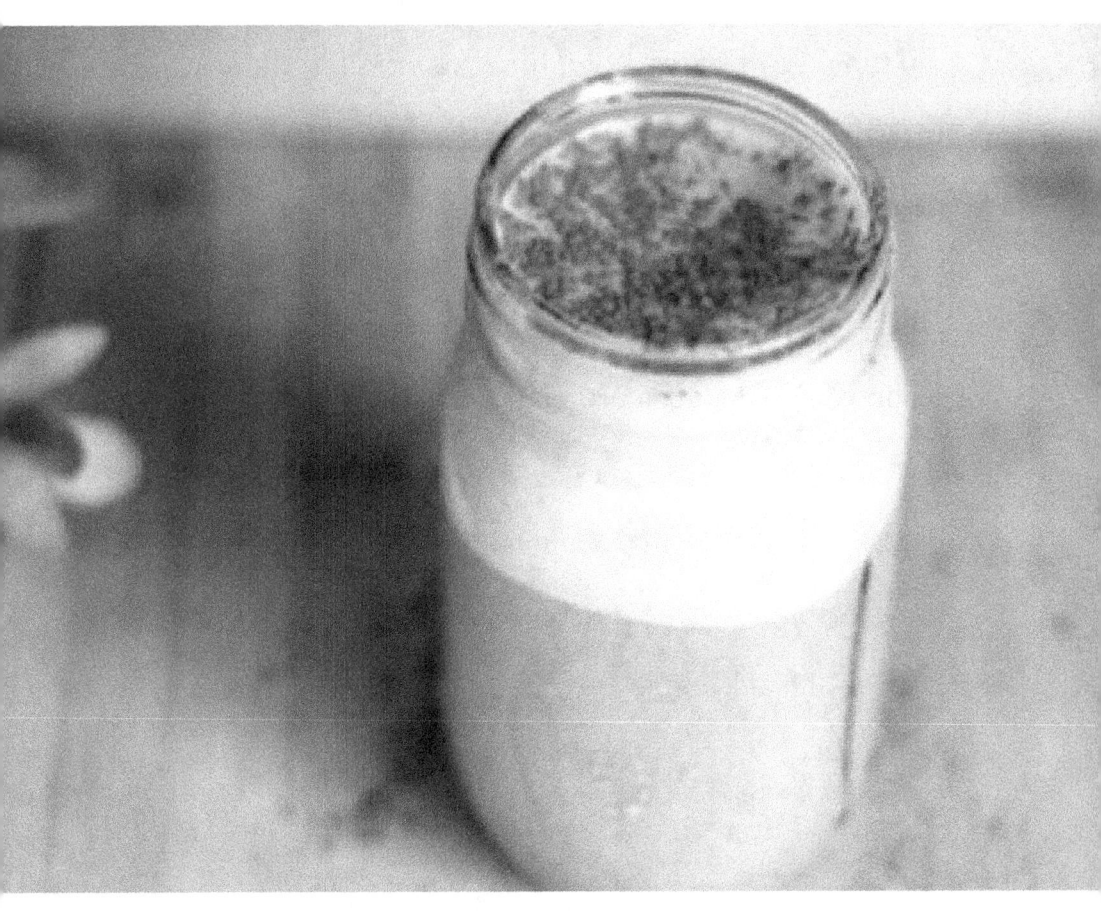

Bulletproof Coffee Egg Latte

Serves 1

Prep time: 12 minutes, Total time: 12 minutes, Calories: 331

Nutritional Information Per Serving: *Proteins: 24g, Carbohydrates: 1g, Fats: 25g*

Ingredients

¼ teaspoon of Ceylon cinnamon

1 scoop vanilla collagen protein

2 pasture-raised eggs

1 -2 teaspoons of Brain Octane oil

1-2 tablespoons of grass fed butter or ghee

8 ounces of black coffee

Directions

Start by adding cinnamon, oil, butter and eggs into the blender.

Add in coffee and blend the mixture on high for 45 seconds.

Add in collagen protein and blend the mixture on low for 5 seconds.

Top the mixture with cinnamon. Serve on a glass and enjoy.

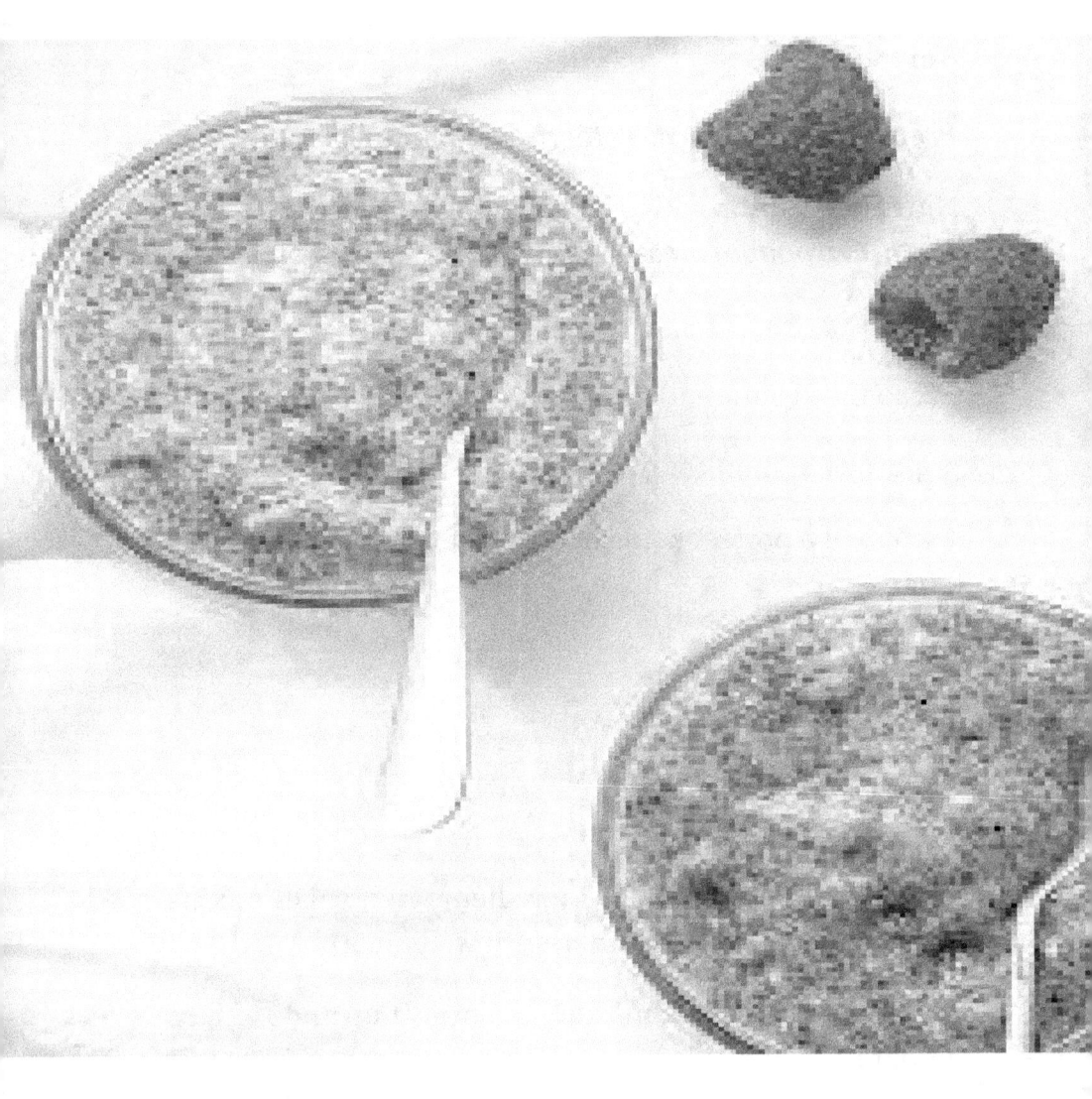

Keto Chia Pudding (Chocolate)

Serves 1

Prep time: 5 minutes, Total time: 5 minutes

Nutritional Information Per Serving: *Calories: 330, Proteins: 18.4g, Carbohydrates: 4.4g, Fats: 20.7g*

Ingredients

Cacao nibs (optional)

3-4 drops of monk fruit sweetener

1 scoop of a perfect keto chocolate keto collagen

1/3 cup of water

¼ cup of almond milk

¼ cup of chia seeds

Directions

Start by adding in all the ingredients in a small mixing bowl. Mix the ingredients together until well incorporated.

Pour the mixture in a mason jar, cover it up and refrigerate for 4 hours.

Serve and enjoy.

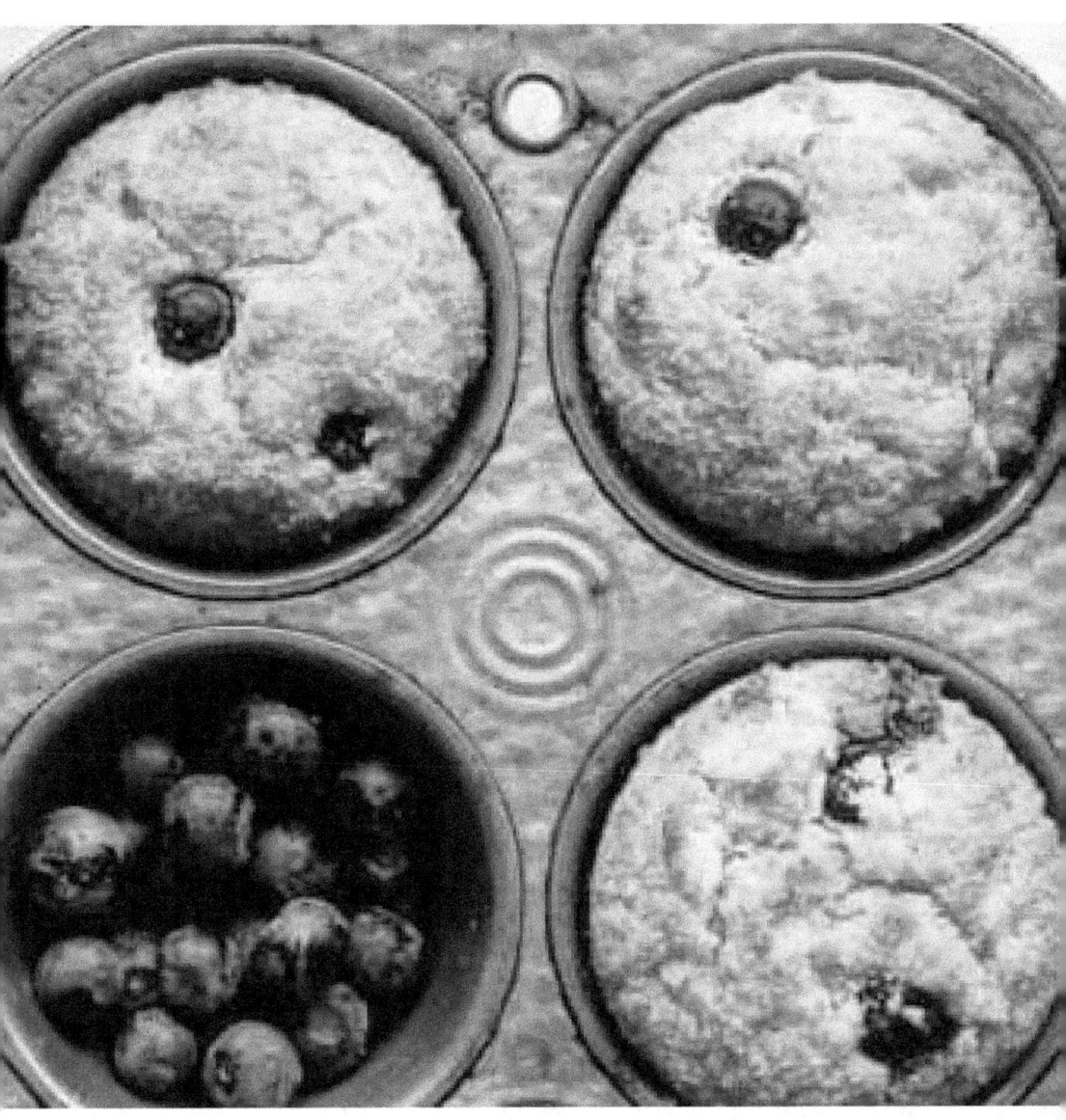

Sugar Free Keto Blueberry Muffins

Serves 12 muffins

Prep time: 20 minutes, Cook time: 25 minutes, Total time: 45 minutes

Nutritional Information Per Serving: *Calories: 247, Proteins: 7.3g, Carbohydrates: 9.3g, Fats: 21.8 g*

Ingredients

2/3 cup of fresh blueberries

2 teaspoons of vanilla extract

½ cup of unsweetened applesauce

3 large eggs at room temperature

7 tablespoons of coconut oil

¾ cup of Monk fruit or any granulated sweetener of your choice

1 teaspoon of baking soda

1 teaspoon of sea salt

1 tablespoon of baking powder

4 tablespoons (32g) of packed coconut flour

3 cups (300g) of almond flour

Directions

Start by preheating your oven to 350 degrees F. Prepare your muffin pan by spraying it with oil.

Prepare the almond mixture: Add baking soda, salt, baking powder, coconut flour and almond flour in a medium sized bowl and mix everything together. Set aside.

Prepare the vanilla mixture: Add in vanilla, applesauce, eggs, and coconut oil and Monk fruit in a large bowl. Use an electric hand mixer to beat everything together until well blended.

Stir in the almond flour mixture into the vanilla mixture together with the blueberries. Mix until everything is well combined. Give the mixture 5 minutes to sit. This enables the coconut flour to start absorbing moisture.

Divide the butter into 12 muffin cavities. Place in the oven and bake for 24-25 minutes or until the muffins turn golden brown and you can insert a toothpick in the center of the muffin and it comes out clean.

Remove from the oven and let it cool for 15 minutes. Run a knife around the edges of the muffins gently to help them loosen up. Let them sit and cool down some more.

Serve in a plate and enjoy them as they are or with a bulletproof coffee.

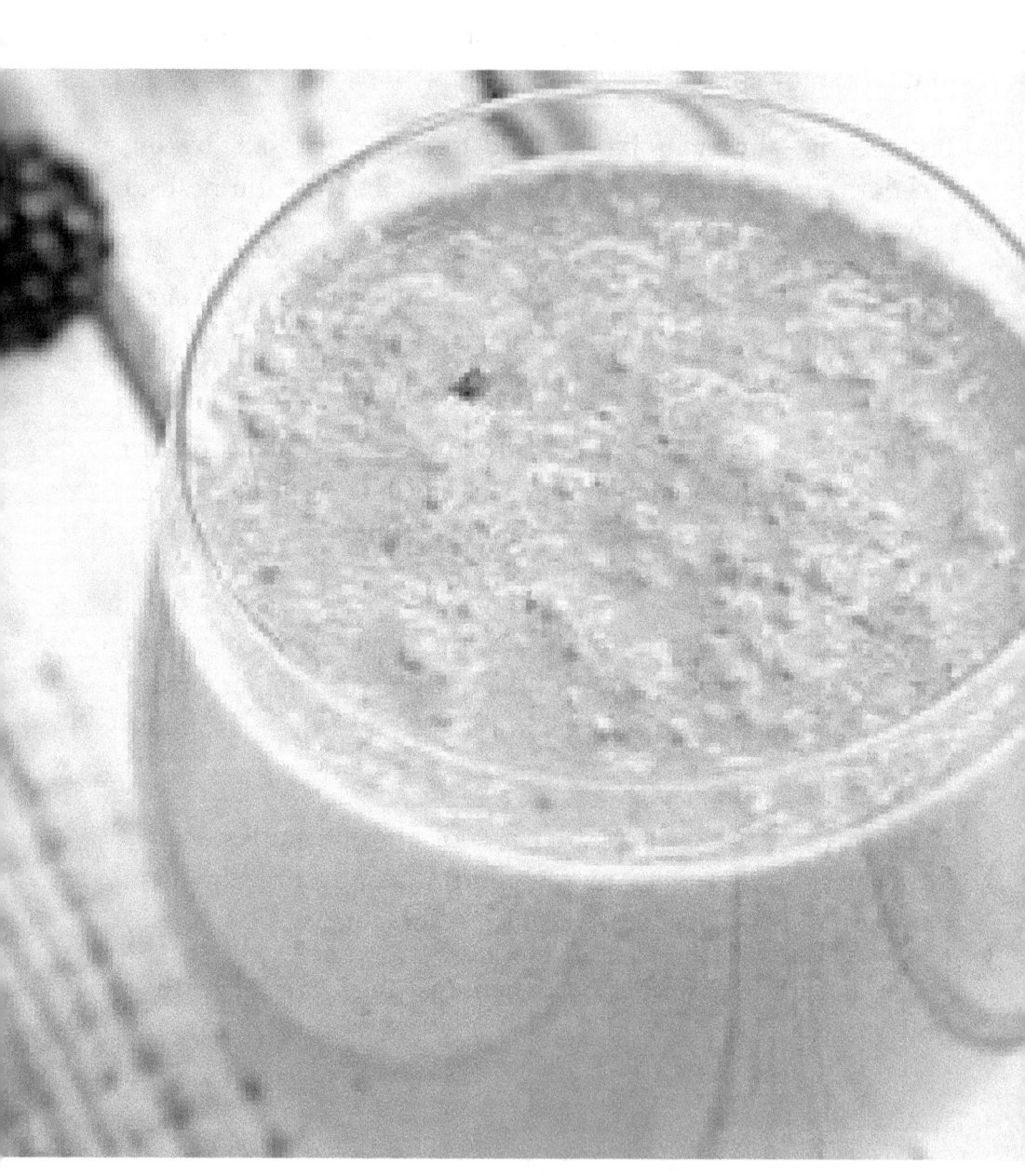

Keto Blackberry Cheesecake Smoothie

Serves 2

Prep time: 5 minutes, Total time: 5 minutes

Nutritional Information Per Serving: *Calories: 515, Proteins: 6.4g, Carbohydrates: 6.7g, Fats: 53g*

Ingredients

½ teaspoon of sugar-free vanilla extract or ¼ teaspoon of pure vanilla powder

1 tablespoon of MCT oil or extra virgin coconut oil

Optional: Keto friendly sweetener e.g. 3-5 drops liquid stevia extract

½ cup of water

¼ cup of heavy whipping cream or 60ml of coconut milk

½ cup of fresh and frozen blackberries.

Directions

Start by placing all the ingredients in a blender.

Pulse the mixture until smooth and frothy.

Pour the mixture in a glass and serve.

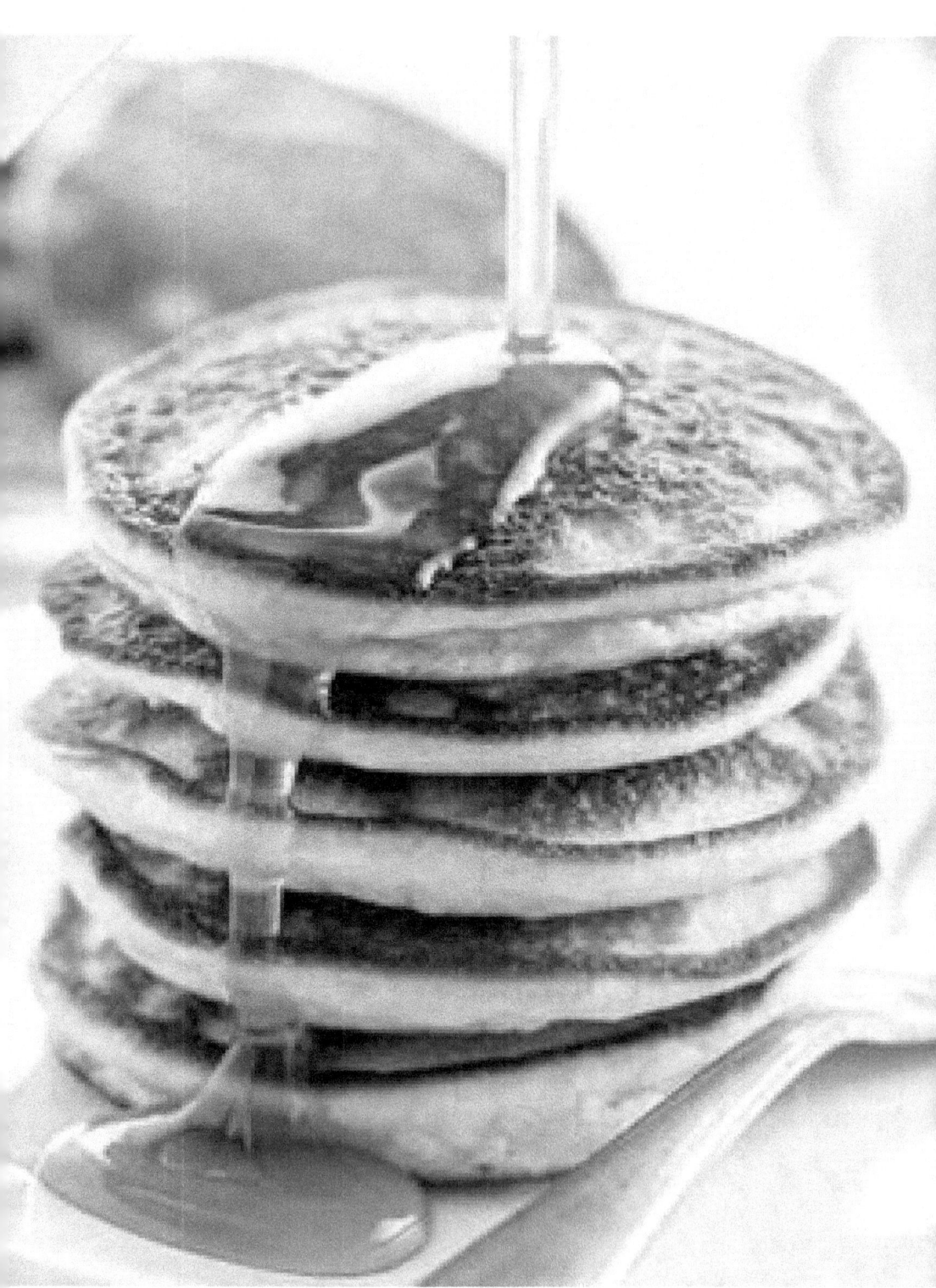

Keto Pancakes

Serves 6

Prep time: 5 minutes, Cook time: 15 minutes, Total time: 20 minutes

Nutritional Information Per Serving: *Calories: 268, Proteins: 9g, Carbohydrates: 6g, Fats: 23 g*

Ingredients

¼ teaspoon of sea salt

Optional: 1 ½ teaspoon of vanilla extract

¼ cup of avocado oil

1/3 cup of unsweetened almond milk

5 large eggs

1 teaspoon of gluten-free baking powder

2-3 tablespoons of Erythritol or any sweetener of your choice

¼ cup of coconut flour

1 cup of blanched almond flour

Directions

In a large bowl, mix all the ingredients together until smooth. The butter should have a typical pancake batter consistency.

Grease your pan with oil and preheat it on the stove over medium-low to medium heat. Pour the batter into the hot pan and form a circle. Cover the pan and let the batter cook until bubbles start to form or for 1 1/2-2 minutes. Flip the pancake and cook until browned or for 1 1/2-2 minutes. Repeat the process until all the batter is used up.

Keto Lunch Recipes

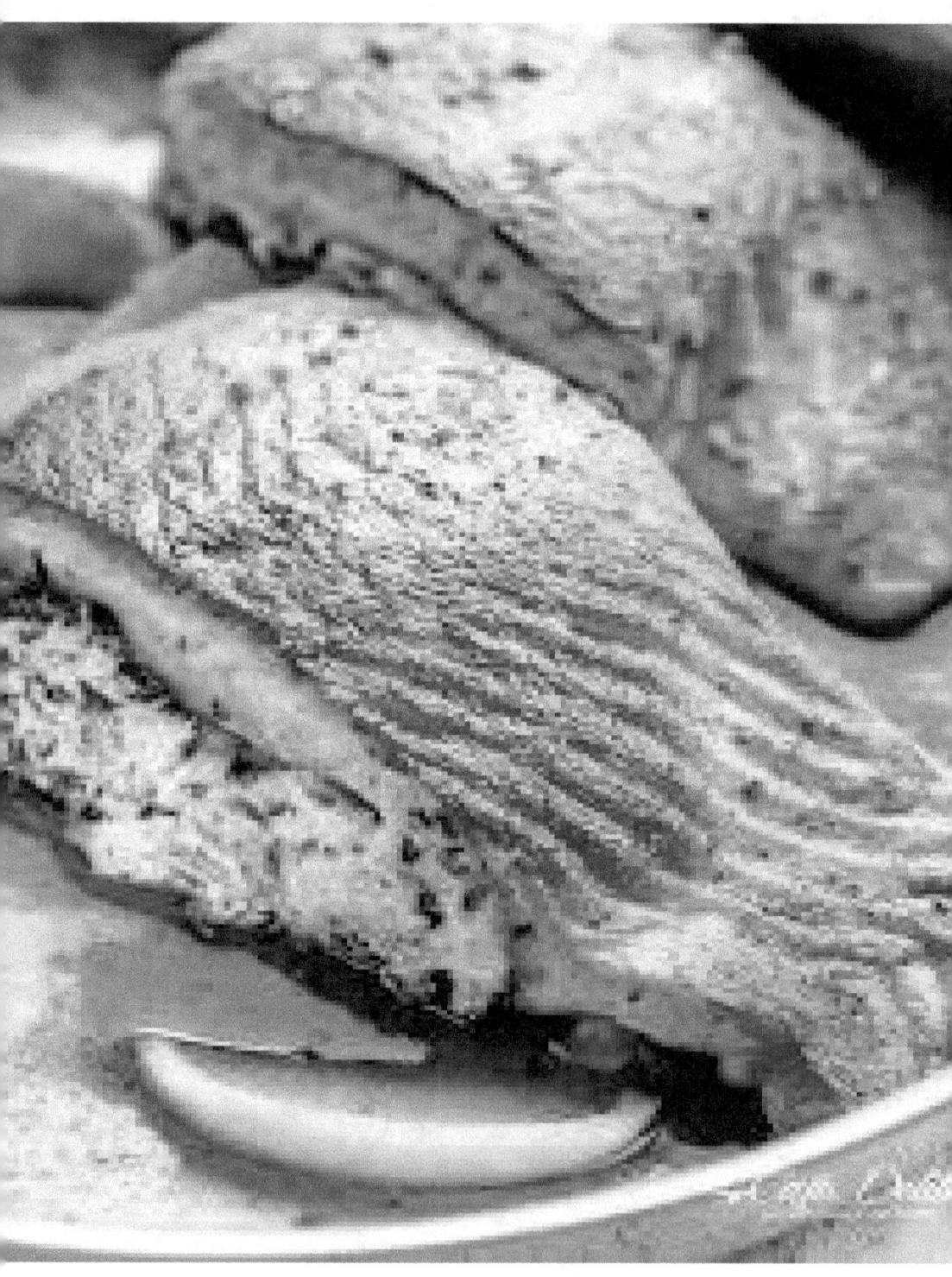

Salmon-Filled Avocados

Serves 2

Prep time: 10 minutes, Total time: 10 minutes

Nutritional Information Per Serving: *Calories: 911, Proteins: 58g, Carbohydrates: 6g, Fats: 71g*

Ingredients

2 tablespoons of lemon juice (optional)

Salt and pepper to taste

¾ cup of mayonnaise or crème fraiche or sour cream

6 ounce of smoked salmon

2 avocados

Directions

Start by cutting your avocados into half and remove the pit.

In the hollow of the avocado, place in a dollop of mayonnaise or crème fraiche and add in the smoked salmon on top.

Season the avocado to taste with salt and pepper and squeeze some lemon juice for extra flavor and to keep the avocado from turning brown.

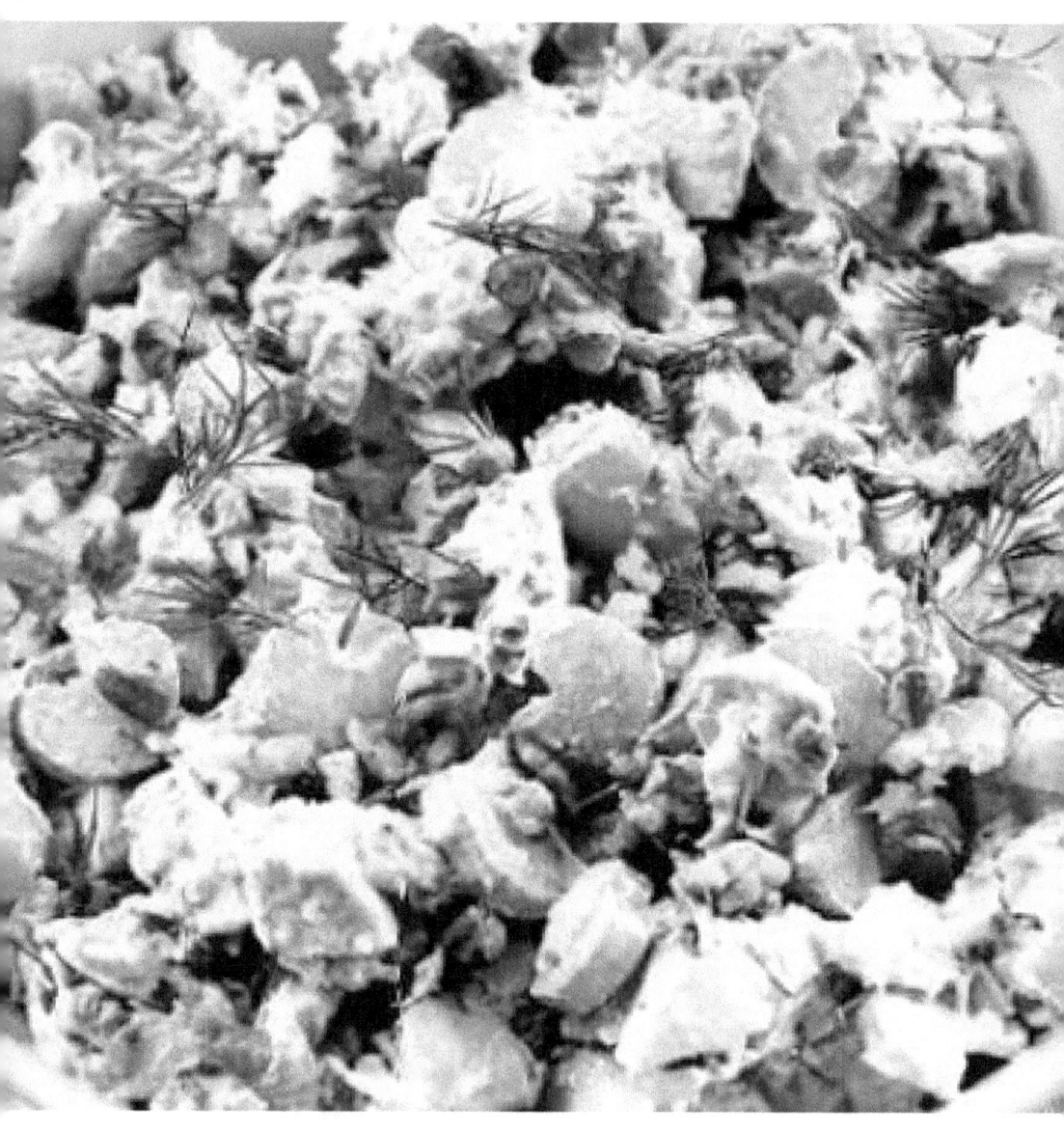

Keto Chicken Salad

Serves 6

Prep time: 1 hr. 15 minutes, Cook time: 15 minutes, Total time: 1 hour 30 minutes

Nutritional Information Per Serving: *Calories: 279, Proteins: 24.8g, Carbohydrates: 0.4g, Fats: 19.4g*

Ingredients

¼ cup of chopped pecans

2 tablespoons of chopped fresh dill

½ teaspoon of pink Himalayan salt

2 teaspoon of brown mustard

½ cup of mayo

3 diced ribs celery

1 ½ lb. chicken breast

Directions

Preheat your oven to 450 degrees F and line a baking sheet with parchment paper.

Place the chicken in the parchment paper and bake it for 15 minutes or until cooked through.

Remove the chicken from the oven, let it cool down and cut it into bite-sized pieces.

Combine a mixture of brown mustard, mayo, celery, salt and chicken into a large bowl.

Toss the ingredients until the chicken is fully coated.

Cover the large bowl with a plastic wrap and refrigerate it for 1-2 hours or until chilled.

Once ready to serve, add chopped pecans, fresh dill and lightly toss. Serve while chilled and enjoy.

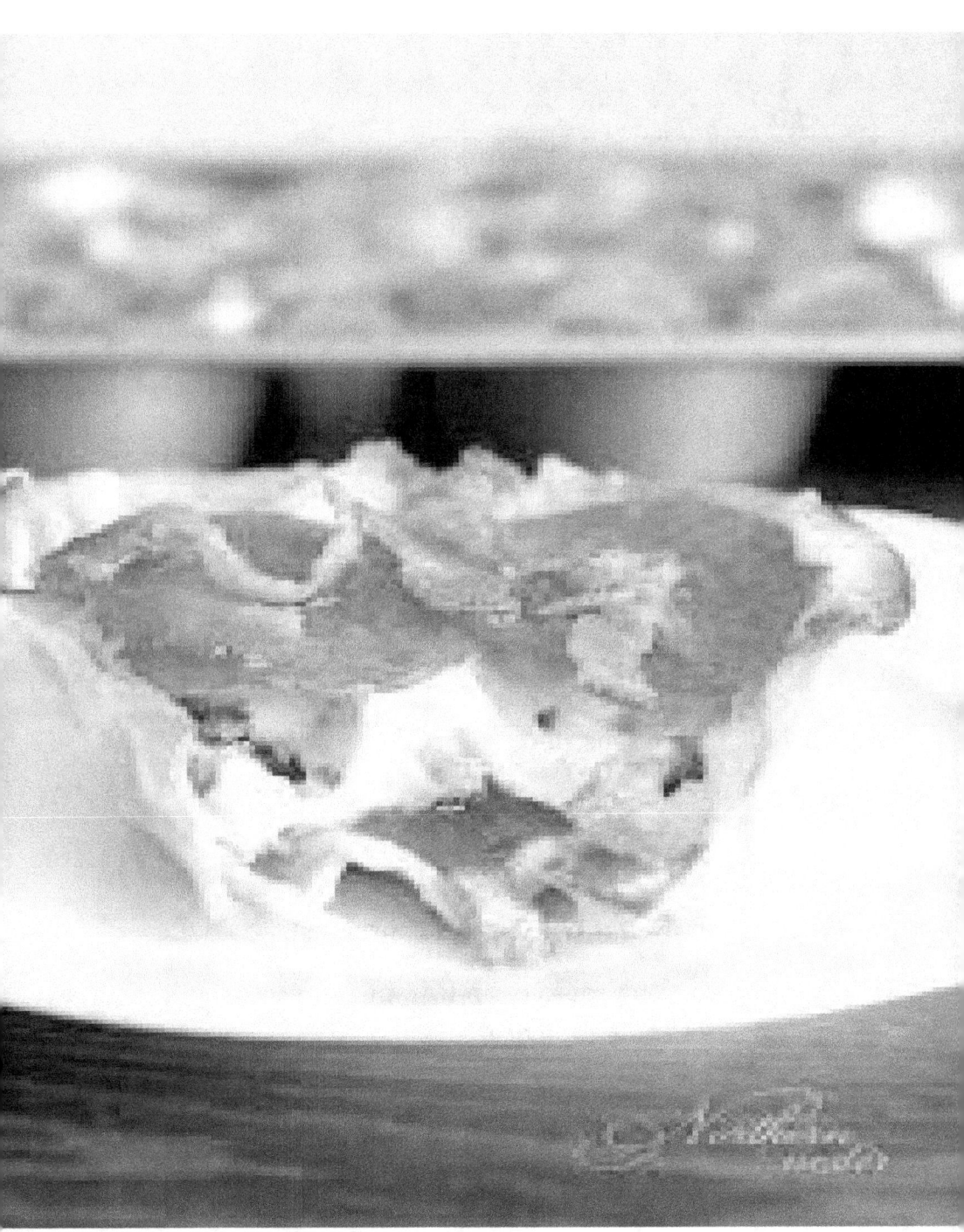

Pizza Cups

Serves 12

Prep time: 15 minutes, Cook time: 11 minutes, Total time: 26 minutes

Nutritional Information Per Serving: *Calories: 266, Proteins: 11g, Carbohydrates: 2.3g, Fats: 10g*

Ingredients

1 cup of cooked and crumbled bacon

24 pepperoni slices

3 cups of grated mozzarella cheese

12 tablespoons of sugar-free pizza sauce

1 lb. bulk Italian sausage

12 deli ham slices

Directions

Preheat your oven to 375 degrees Fahrenheit.

Then brown your sausage and drain the excess grease in a frying pan, over medium heat.

Line 12 cups of muffin tins with ham slices. Add in sausage, then pizza sauce, followed by mozzarella cheese, and then pepperoni slices and finally bacon crumbles in all the muffin tins and in that order.

Place the muffin tins in the oven and bake for 10 minutes at 375 degrees Fahrenheit. Broil the pizza for 1 minute or until it browns and until the cheese bubbles. The edges of the meat toppings should look crispy.

Transfer the pizza cups from the muffin tins to a paper towel. This will prevent the bottom of the pizza from getting wet.

Serve and enjoy. You can also refrigerate to eat later.

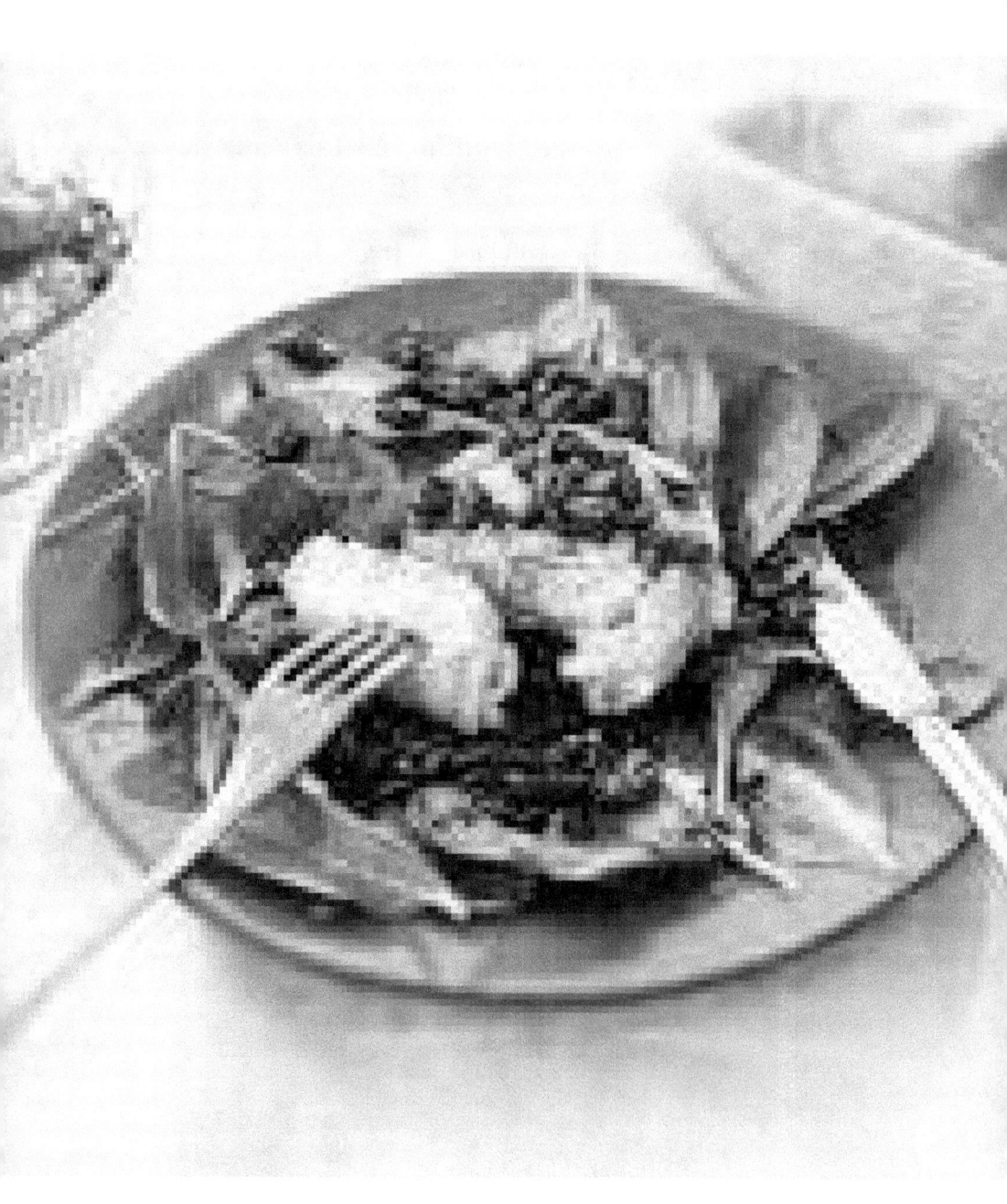

Goat Cheese Salad With Balsamico Butter

Serves 2

Prep time: 5 minutes, Cook time: 20 minutes, Total time: 25 minutes

Nutritional Information Per Serving: *Calories: 824, Proteins: 37g, Carbohydrates: 3g, Fats: 73g*

Ingredients

3 ounce of baby spinach

1 tablespoon of balsamic vinegar

2 ounces of butter

¼ cup of pumpkin seeds

10 ounces of goat cheese

Directions

Preheat your oven to 200 degrees Celsius.

Grease a baking dish and place in slices of goat cheese. Put the baking dish in the oven and bake for 10 minutes.

As the goat cheese bakes, you can be toasting your pumpkin seeds. In a dry frying pan that is over fairly high temperature, toast the pumpkin seeds until they color and start to pop up.

Lower the heat to low, add butter and let the seeds simmer until they turn golden brown and produce a pleasant nutty scent. Add in balsamic vinegar and let the mixture boil for a few minutes. Turn the heat off.

On a large plate, spread out your baby spinach and place the cheese on top of it. Add in the Balsamico butter and enjoy.

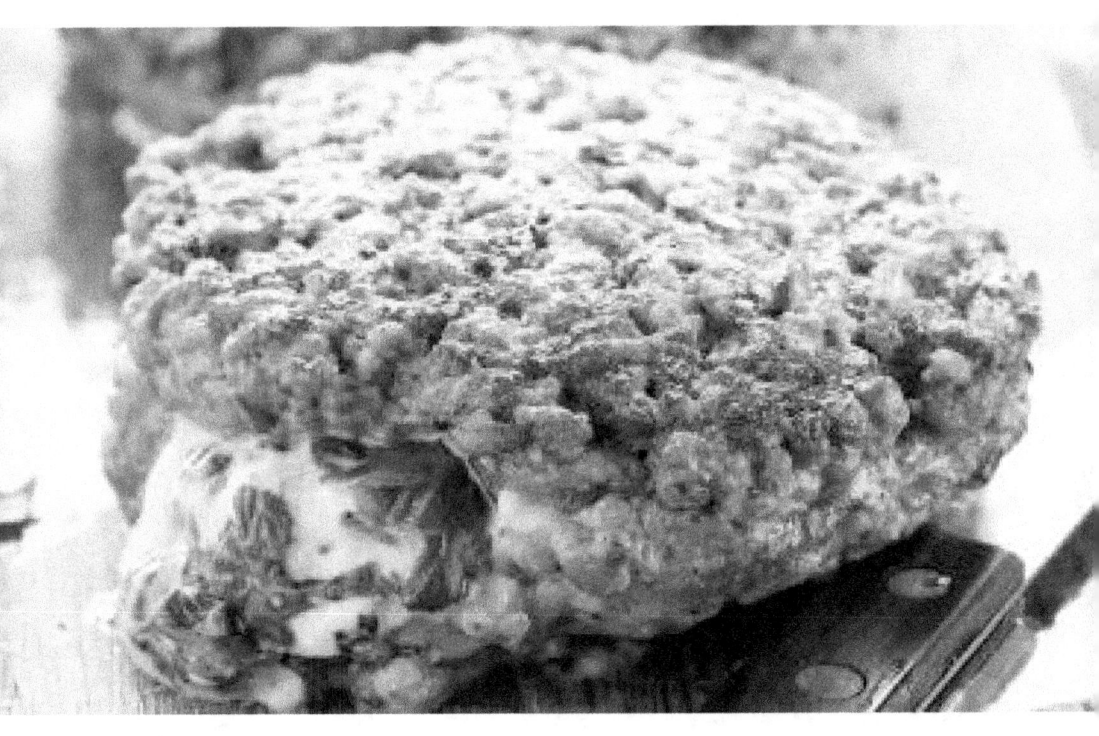

Keto Spinach Mozzarella Stuffed Burgers

Serves 4

Prep time: 15 minutes, Cook time: 20 minutes, Total time: 35 minutes

Nutritional Information Per Serving: *Calories: 414, Proteins: 36g, Carbohydrates: 1g, Fats: 29 g*

Ingredients

2 tablespoons of grated Parmesan cheese

½ cup of shredded mozzarella cheese

2 cups of firmly packed fresh spinach

¾ teaspoon of ground black pepper

1 teaspoon of salt

1 ½ lbs. of ground chuck

Directions

Start by combining a mix of ground beef, salt and pepper in a medium sized bowl.

Use dampened hands to scoop about 1/3 cup of the beef mixture and shape them into 8 patties. The patties should be ½ inch thick. Place them in the refrigerator.

Place your spinach in a saucepan that is over medium-high heat. Cover the saucepan and let it cook until wilted or for 2 minutes. Drain the spinach and let it cool. Pick the spinach with your hands and squeeze them to remove as much liquid as possible.

Place the spinach in a cutting board and chop them off. Transfer the spinach into a bowl. Then stir in the parmesan and mozzarella cheese. Scoop ¼ cup of spinach mix and stuff it in the center of four patties and then cover each one of them using the other four patties. Seal the edges of the patties by pressing the edges firmly together.

Cup each of the patties using your hands to round out the edges. Press on top of each patty to flatten them slightly into one thick patty.

Heat your grill pan to medium-high. Lightly oil the grill gates if you are using an outdoor grill.

Grill your burgers for 5-6 minutes on each side. Serve and enjoy.

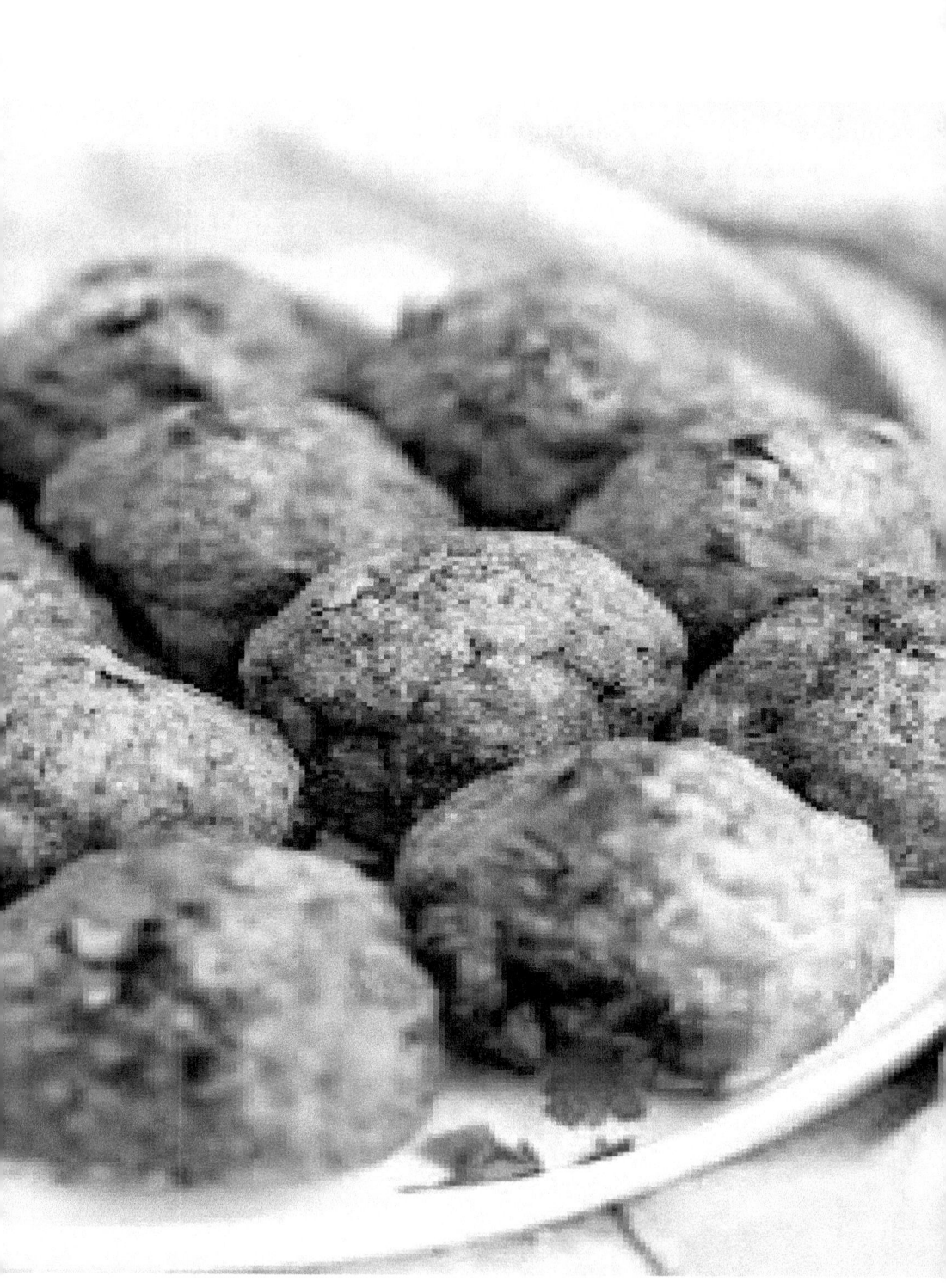

Keto Meatballs

Serves 8-10

Prep time: 5 minutes, Cook time: 20 minutes, Total time: 25 minutes

Nutritional Information Per Serving: *Calories: 153, Proteins: 12.2g, Carbohydrates: 0.7g, Fats: 10.9g*

Ingredients

½ teaspoon of salt

1 teaspoon of black pepper

1 tablespoon of minced garlic

½ cup of shredded mozzarella

½ cup of grated parmesan

1 large egg

1 lb. of ground beef

Directions

Start by preheating your oven to 400 degrees F. Line your baking sheet with parchment paper.

Use your hands to combine all the ingredients in a mixing bowl. Knead the mixture together until it's well-incorporated.

Use your hands to form equal sized meatballs from the mixture you have just made. Place them on the baking sheet.

Place the baking sheet in the oven and bake for 18-20 minutes.

Remove from the oven and let it cool.

Serve and enjoy.

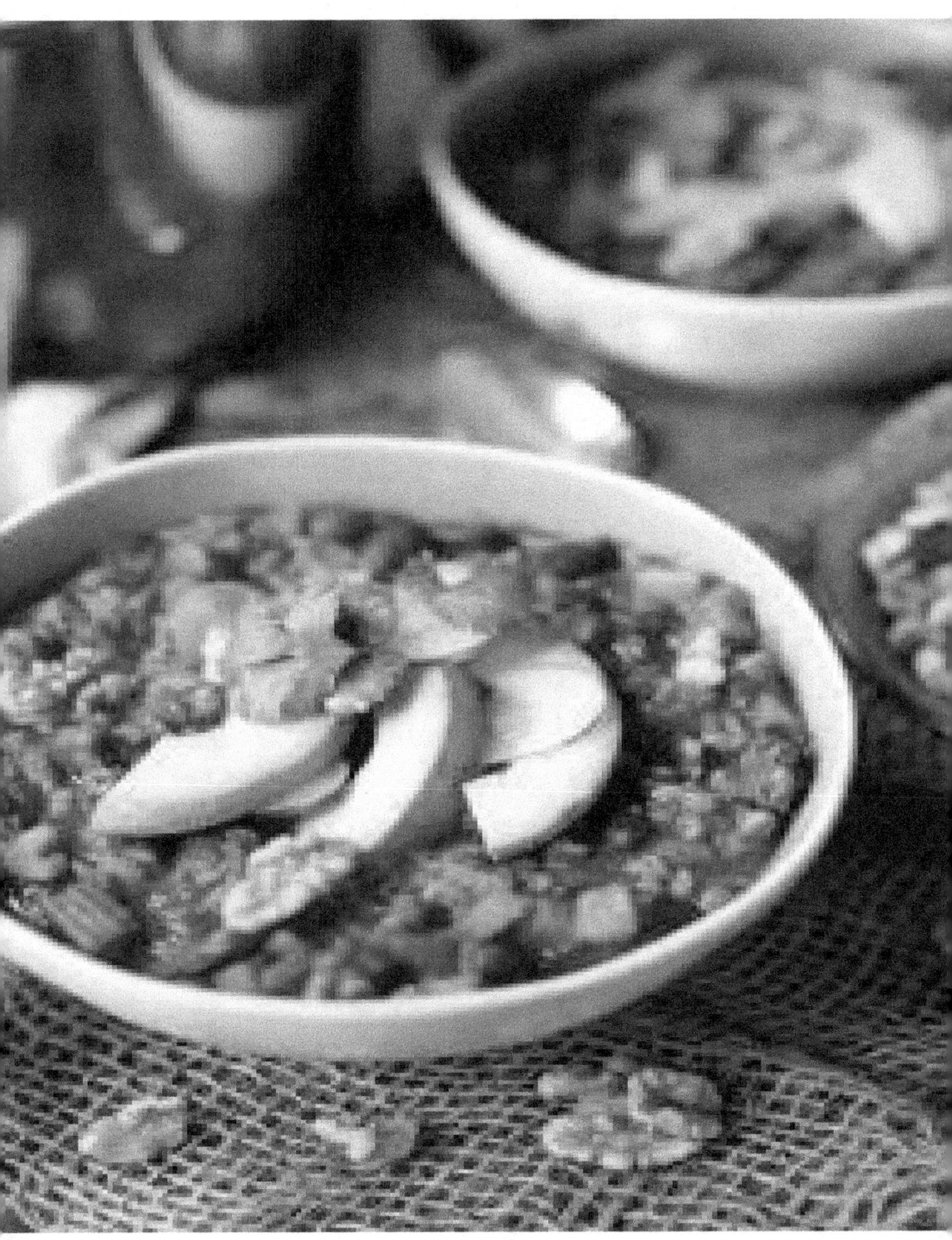

Vegan Walnut Chili

Serves 6-8

Prep time: 10 minutes, Cook time: 31 minutes, Total time: 41 minutes

Nutritional Information Per Serving: *Calories: 353, Proteins: 6g, Carbohydrates: 1g, Fats: 15g*

Ingredients

Salt and pepper

1 tablespoon of unsweetened cocoa powder

1 cup of minced raw walnuts

2 ½ cups of crumbled soy meat

½ cup of coconut milk

3 cups of water

1 15 ounce can of diced tomatoes

1 ½ tablespoons of tomato paste

8 ounces of cremini mushrooms

2 diced zucchini

2 finely diced green bell peppers

2 peppers large chipotle in adobo

1 ½ teaspoons of smoked paprika

4 teaspoons of ground cumin

2 teaspoons of chili powder

1 ½ teaspoons of ground cinnamon

2 cloves garlic, minced

5 finely diced stalks of celery

2 tablespoons of extra virgin olive oil

To serve

2 tablespoons of sliced radishes

1 avocado sliced

2 tablespoons of fresh cilantro leaves

Directions

Start by oiling a large pot and heating it over medium heat. Add in celery and let it cook for 4 minutes. Add in paprika, cumin, chili powder, cinnamon, and garlic and stir them for two minutes or until fragrant.

Add in mushrooms, zucchini and ball peppers and let the mixture cook for 5 minutes.

Add in cocoa powder, walnuts, soy meat, coconut milk, water, tomatoes, tomato paste and chipotle. Reduce heat to medium low and let the food simmer for 20-25 minutes or until the mixture is thick and the vegetable is soft.

Season the food with salt and pepper to taste and top the mixture with cilantro, radishes and avocado.

Serve and enjoy.

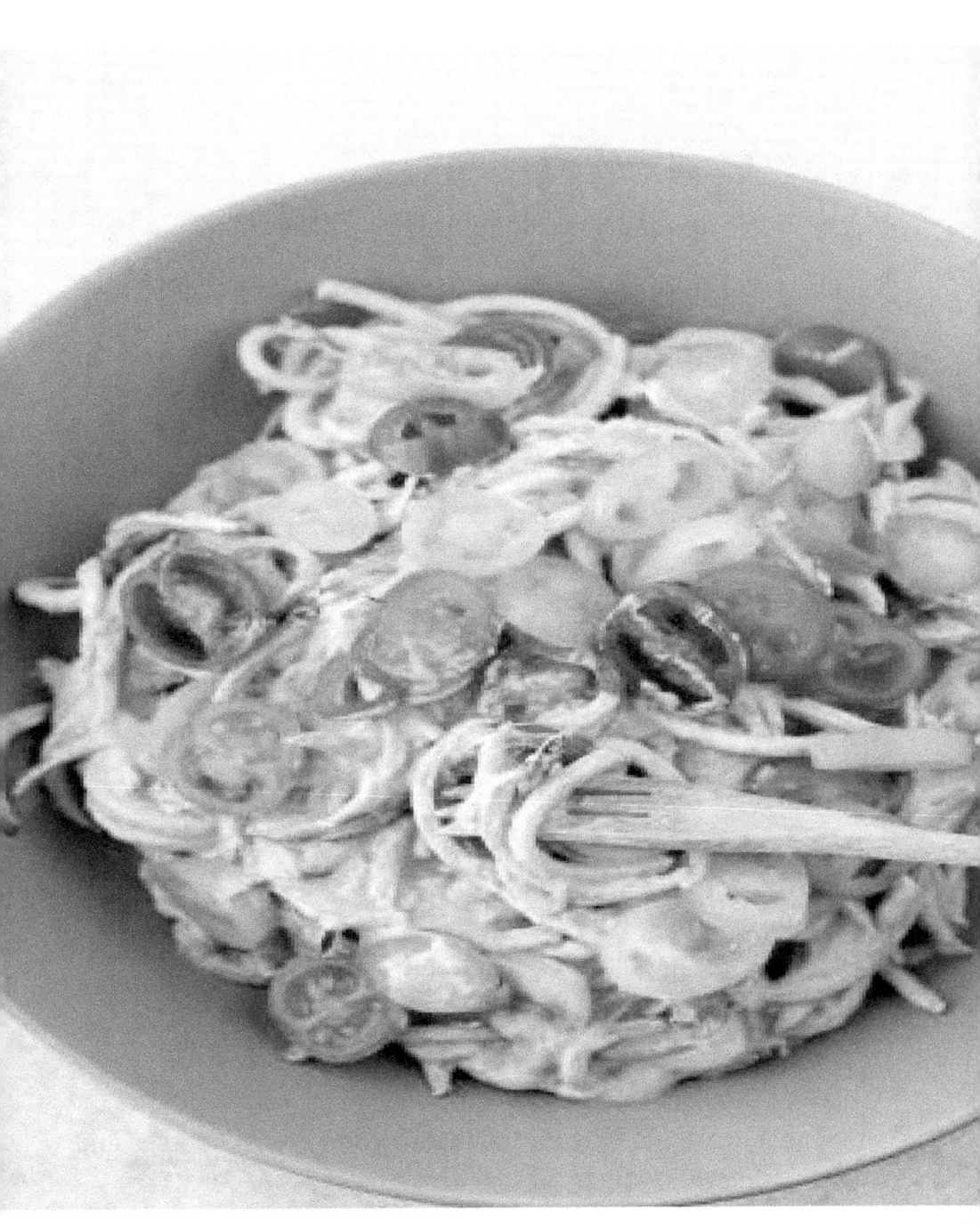

Zucchini Noodles With Avocado Sauce

Serves 2

Prep time: 10 minutes, Total time: 10 minutes

Nutritional Information Per Serving: *Calories: 313, Proteins: 6.8g, Carbohydrates: 18.7g, Fats: 26.8g*

Ingredients

12 sliced cherry tomatoes

1 avocado

2 tablespoons of lemon juice

4 tablespoons of pine nuts

1/3 cup of water

1 ¼ cups of basil

1 zucchini

Directions

Make the zucchini noodles using the spiralizer or a peeler.

In a blender, add in all the other ingredients except for the cherry tomatoes. Blend until smooth.

Use a mixing bowl to combine the avocado sauce, noodles and cherry tomatoes. Mix until well combined.

Serve and enjoy.

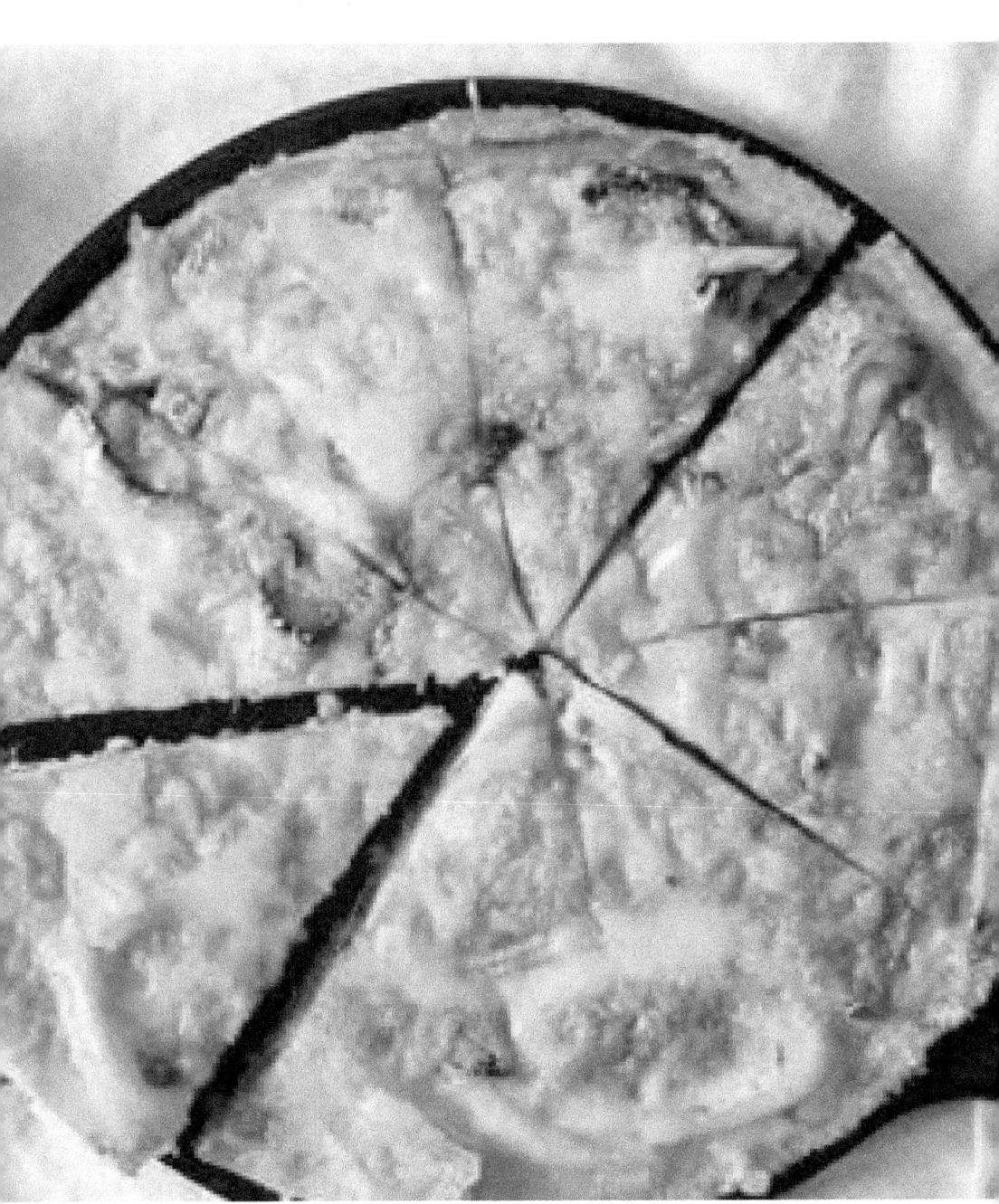

Turkey Sausage Frittata

Serves 8

Prep time: 10 minutes, Cook time: 30 minutes, Total time: 40 minutes

Nutritional Information Per Serving: *Calories: 240, Proteins: 16.7g, Carbohydrates: 5.5g, Fats: 16.7g*

Ingredients

2 teaspoons of Kerry Gold butter

1 teaspoon of black pepper

1 teaspoon of pink Himalayan salt

Optional: 2 ounce of shredded Tillamook cheddar

1 cup of lactose free sour cream

12 eggs

2 bell peppers

12 ounces of ground breakfast sausage turkey

Directions

Preheat your oven to 350 degrees Fahrenheit.

In a blender, crack in all your eggs. Add in salt, pepper and sour cream. Blend on high for 30 seconds and set the mixture aside.

Place a large skillet over medium heat. Add the butter once the pan is hot.

Prepare your bell peppers by slicing them into strips and add them to the skillet. Sauté the peppers for 6 minutes or until they are tender and brown; remove from the skillet.

Prepare the turkey by adding the turkey sausage in the skillet and stir as you break up the meat- Do that for 8 minutes or until the meat is browned. Flatten the turkey by pressing it down. Add in the peppers in an even manner and pour the egg mix on top.

Put the skillet in the oven and bake for 30 minutes. If you want your frittata to have cheese, sprinkle some cheese on top of the frittata immediately you remove it from the oven.

Serve and enjoy.

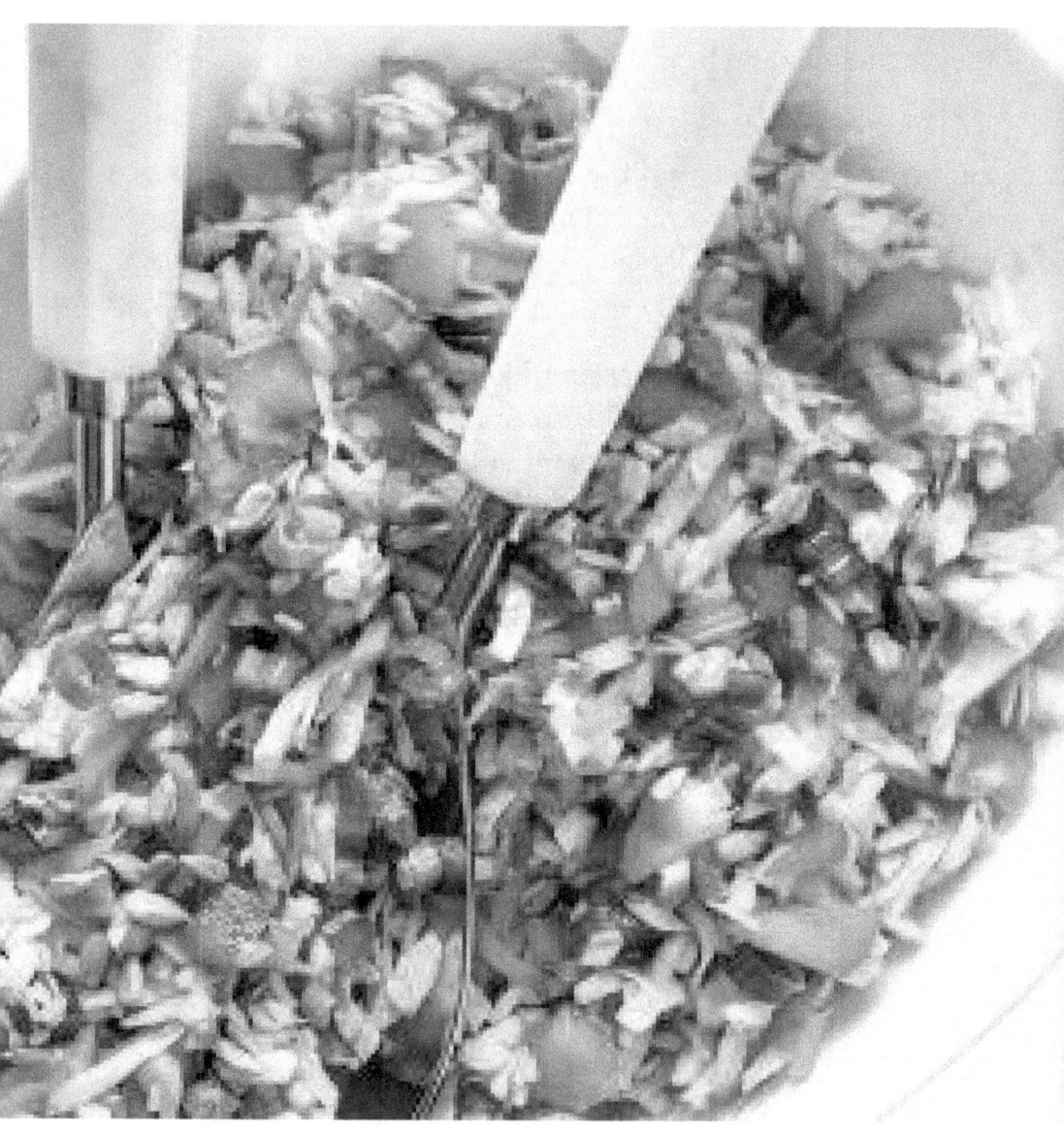

Asian Cabbage Salad

Serves 6

Prep time: 5 minutes, Total time: 5 minutes

Nutritional Information Per Serving: *Calories: 120, Proteins: 2g, Carbohydrates: 6g, Fats: 9g*

Ingredients

Oriental salad

¼ cup of sunflower seeds

2 medium green onions, sliced

1 medium bell pepper, diced

14 ounces of coleslaw mix

Oriental salad dressing

½ teaspoon of salt

½ teaspoon of garlic powder

2 teaspoons of toasted sesame oil

1 tablespoon of white wine vinegar

3 tablespoons of coconut aminos

2 tablespoons of olive oil

Directions

Whisk together all the dressing ingredients in a large bowl.

Add in all the salad ingredients and toss everything together until the salad is well-coated.

Serve and enjoy. Or refrigerate to eat later.

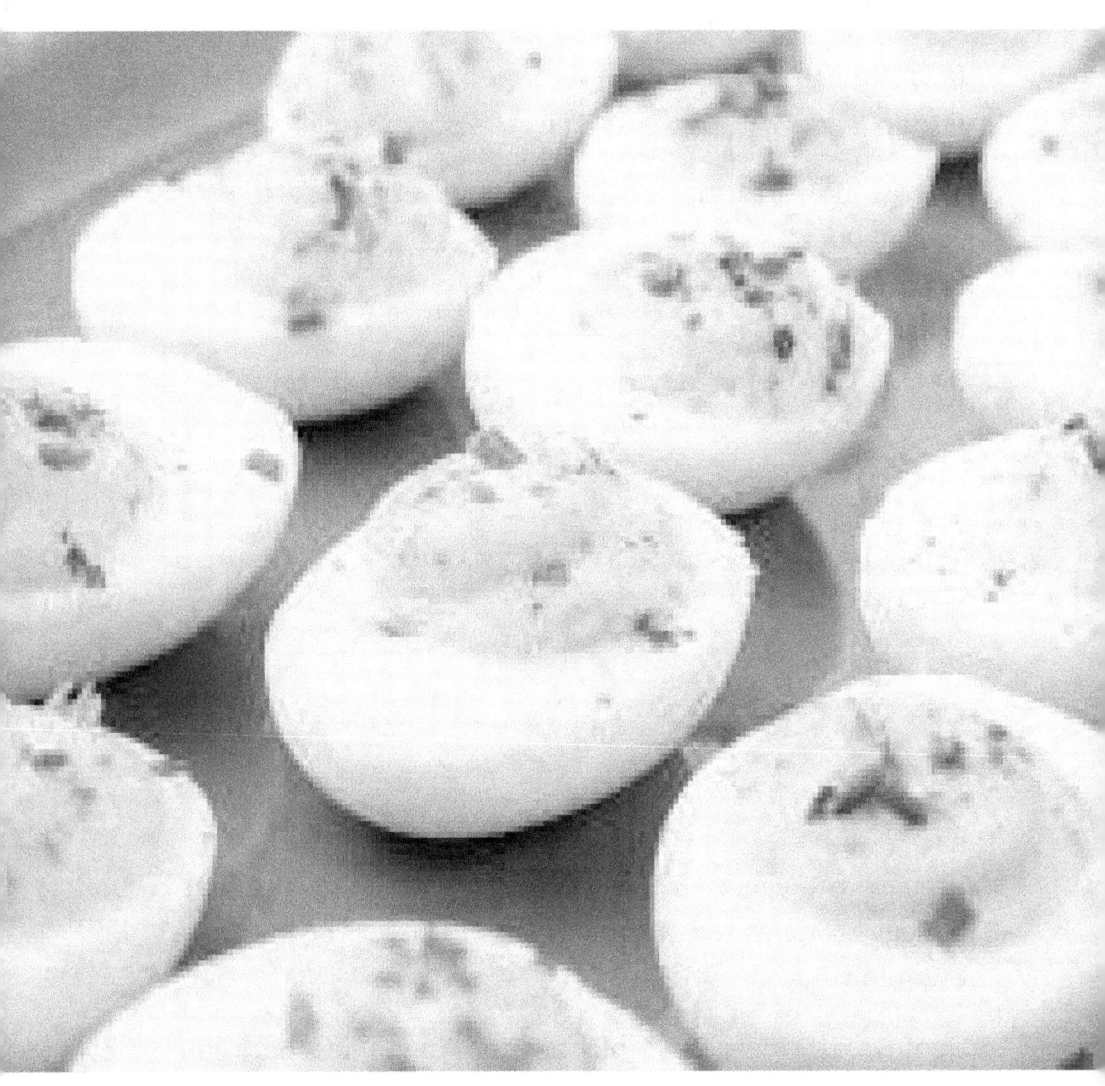

Deviled Eggs

Serves 4

Prep time: 10 minutes, Cook time: 10 minutes, Total time: 20 minutes

Nutritional Information Per Serving: *Calories: 163, Proteins: 7g, Carbohydrates: 0.5g, Fats: 15g*

Ingredients

8 peeled and cooked shrimps or strips of smoked salmon

Fresh dill

1 pinch of herbal salt

¼ cup of mayonnaise

1 teaspoon of Tabasco

4 eggs

Directions

Prepare the eggs: Use a pot that is over medium heat to boil the eggs. The water in the pot should cover the eggs. Hard boil them for 8-10 minutes

Remove the eggs and place them in an ice bath for a few minutes before you can start peeling them.

Cut the eggs into half and scoop out the yolks. Transfer the halved egg whites on a plate.

Place the egg yolks in a bowl and mash them using a fork. Add in Tabasco, homemade mayonnaise and herbal salt. Mix until well combined.

Scoop the yolk mixture and place it on the hollow part of each egg white. Top it off with a piece of shrimp on each egg white.

Decorate it with the dill and serve.

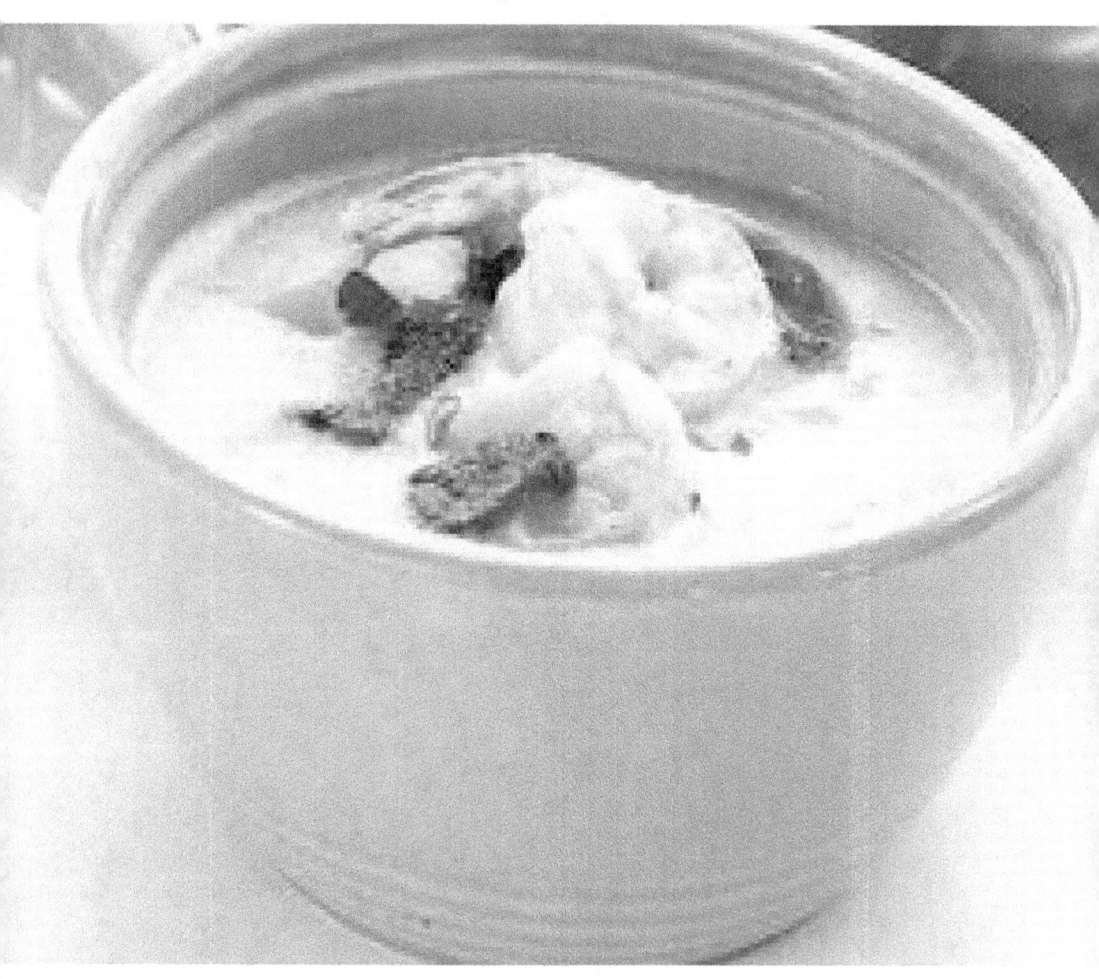

Keto Shrimp And Bacon Chowder

Serves 6

Prep time: 5 minutes, Cook time: 25 minutes, Total time: 30 minutes

Nutritional Information Per Serving: *Calories: 391, Proteins: 16.5g, Carbohydrates: 5.6g, Fats: 31.9g*

Ingredients

Salt and pepper

½ teaspoon of Cajun seasoning

1 pound of shrimp deveined and peeled (tails on or off)

1 cup of heavy whipping cream

2 cups of chicken broth

Chopped parsley for garnish

2 cloves of garlic, minced

½ cup of chopped onion

1 medium turnip that is cut into ½ inch cubes

6 slices of chopped bacon

Directions

Start by preparing the bacon: Cook the bacon in a large pot over medium heat. Let it cook until crisp. Transfer the bacon to a paper towel using a slotted spoon. Let it drain as you leave the bacon fat in the pan.

Add onion and turnip to the pot with the bacon fat and let the onion sauté for 5 minutes or until tender. Stir in the garlic. Let it cook for a minute or so or until fragrant. Pour the chicken broth in and simmer for 10 minutes or until the turnip becomes tender.

Stir the cream and the shrimp in and let the food simmer for 3 minutes or so or until the shrimp turns pink and is well cooked. Add in Cajun seasoning and season the food with salt and pepper to taste.

Serve the food in a plate and garnish it with bacon and chopped parsley.

Serve and enjoy.

Keto Dinner Recipes

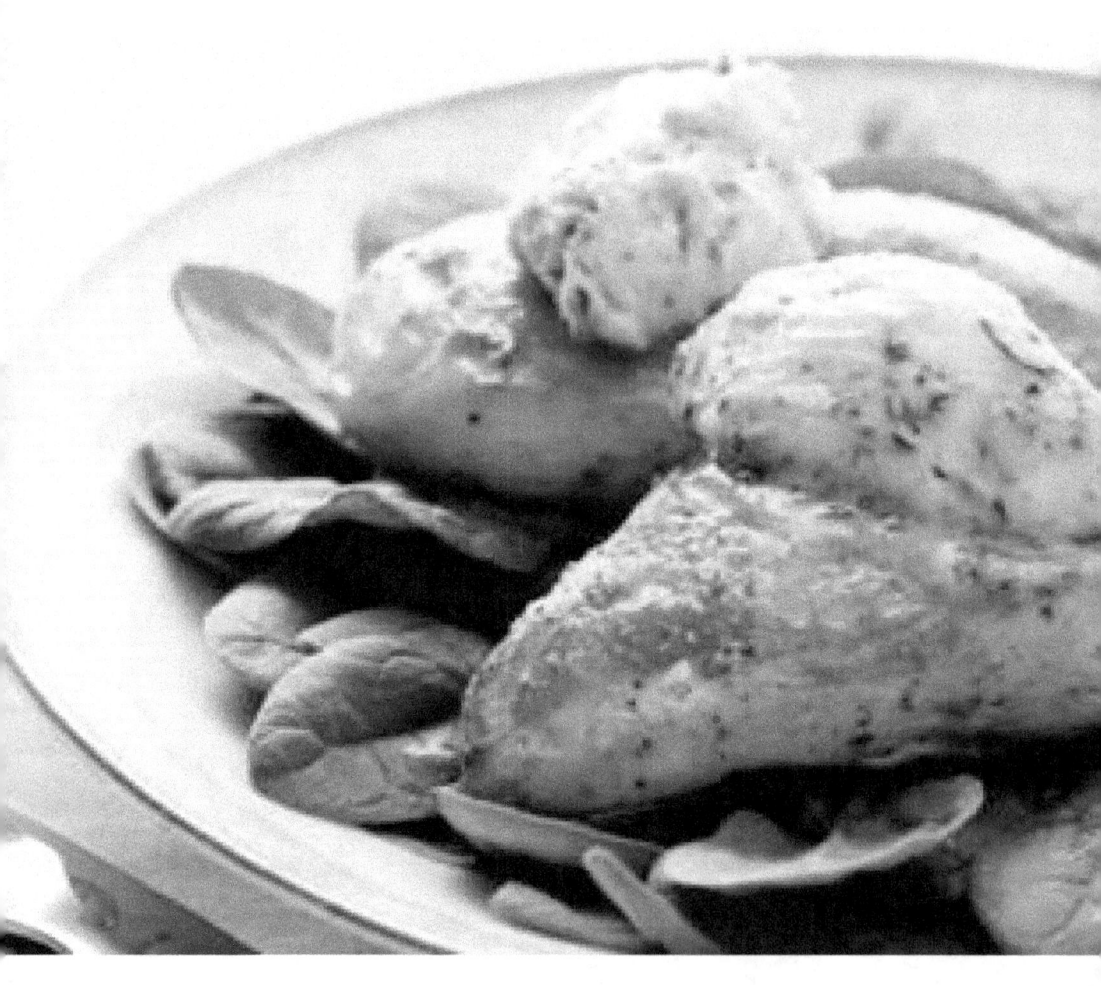

Keto Chicken With Herb

Serves 4

Prep time: 5 minutes, Cook time: 10 minutes, Total time: 15 minutes

Nutritional Information Per Serving: *Calories: 898, Proteins: 63g, Carbohydrates: 2g, Fats: 70g*

Ingredients

Herb butter

½ teaspoon of salt

1 teaspoon of lemon juice

¼ cup of fresh parsley that is finely chopped

½ teaspoon of garlic powder

1 garlic clove

6 ounce of butter at room temperature

Fried chicken

Salt and pepper

4 chicken breasts

3 tablespoons of butter or olive oil

Serving

8 ounces of leafy greens like kale or baby spinach

Directions

Start by preparing the herb butter: Add all the herb butter ingredients in a small bowl and mix everything thoroughly. Let the mix sit.

Prepare the chicken: Melt the butter in a large frying pan over medium heat. As the butter melts, season the chicken with salt and pepper. Place the chicken on the pan and let it fry in butter until the meat thermometer reads 75 degrees Celsius or until the filets are cooked through. You should lower the temperature towards the end to avoid having dry chicken.

Transfer the fried chicken to a bed of leafy greens and add in a generous amount of herb butter on top. Enjoy.

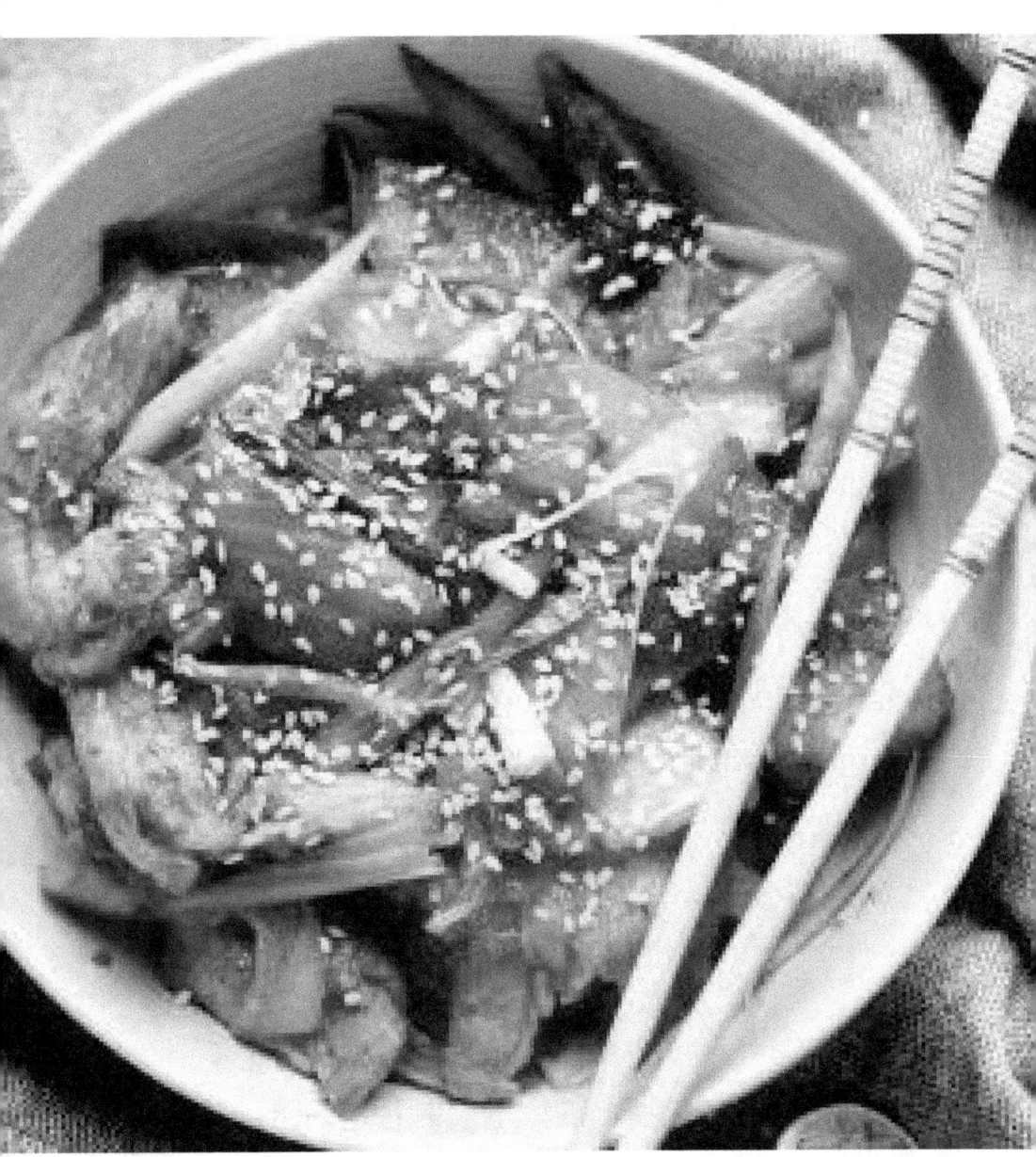

Pork Belly And Stir Fry Kimchi

Serves 3

Prep time: 5 minutes, Cook time: 15 minutes, Total time: 20 minutes

Nutritional Information Per Serving: *Calories: 458, Proteins: 10g, Carbohydrates: 10g, Fats: 42g*

Ingredients

Optional: 1 tablespoon of sesame seeds

1 stalk of green onion

1 lb. of kimchi

1 tablespoon of natural brewed rice wine

1 tablespoon of naturally brewed tamari or soy sauce

300 grams of naturally-raised pork belly

Directions

Start by preparing the pork belly: Slice the pork belly into thin slices. Marinate the slices in rice wine and tamari/soy sauce for about 10 minutes.

Cut your kimchi into 1 inch sizes if it was not pre-cut.

Stir fry the marinated pork belly using a heavy bottom pan that is over medium heat. Fry the pork for 5-10 minutes or until the pork browns. At this point, some fat will be cooking out of the pork belly.

Add kimchi into the pan and stir fry the mixture for a further 2 minutes. This will mix the flavor of kimchi and pork. Turn the heat off.

Slice the green onions and add them into the stir fry. If you prefer, you can sprinkle the sesame seeds. Serve and enjoy.

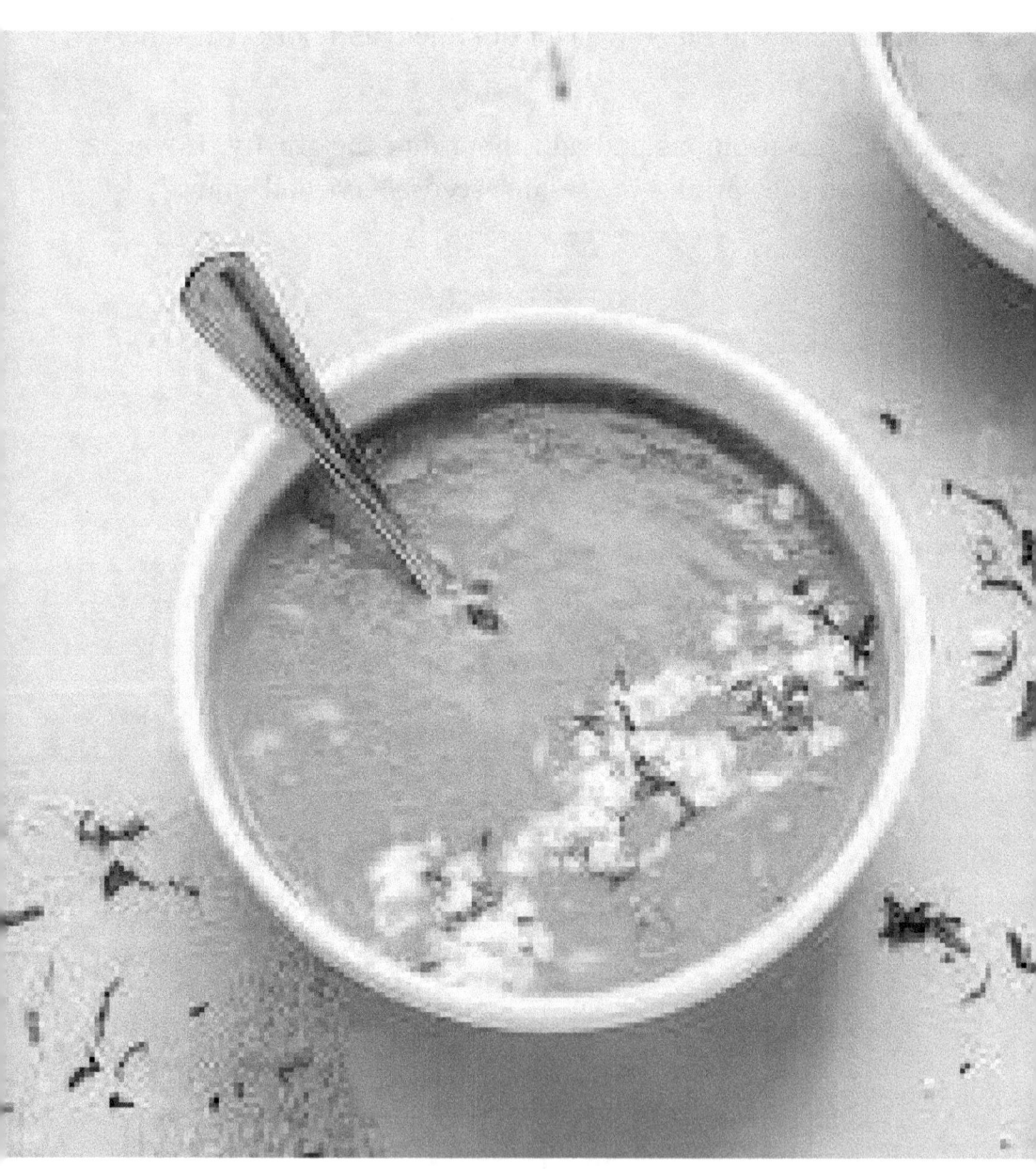

Tomato Feta Soup

Serves 6

Prep time: 5 minutes, Cook time: 25 minutes, Total time: 30 minutes

Nutritional Information Per Serving: *Calories: 170, Proteins: 4g, Carbohydrates: 10g, Fats: 13g*

Ingredients

2/3 cup of crumbled feta cheese

1/3 cup of heavy cream

3 cups of water

Optional: 1 teaspoon of erythritol/sugar or honey

10 tomatoes that are chopped seeded and skinned

Optional: 1 tablespoon of tomato paste

1 teaspoon of dried basil

½ teaspoon of dried oregano

Optional: 1 teaspoon of pesto sauce

1/8 teaspoon of black pepper

½ teaspoon of salt

2 cloves of garlic

¼ cup of chopped onion

2 tablespoons of olive oil or butter

Directions

In a large pot (Dutch oven) placed over medium heat, heat olive oil. Add in onions and cook it for about 2 minutes as you stir it frequently. Add garlic and cook it for 1 minute.

Add water, tomato paste, basil, oregano, pesto, pepper, salt and tomatoes. Bring the mixture to a boil and then reduce the heat for it to simmer. Add sweetener. Let the soup cook for 20 minutes on medium heat or until the tomato is tender.

Use an immersion blender to blend the soup until smooth. Add in feta cheese and cream. Let the soup cook for a further 1 minute. Taste the soup and season appropriately using salt.

Serve while warm.

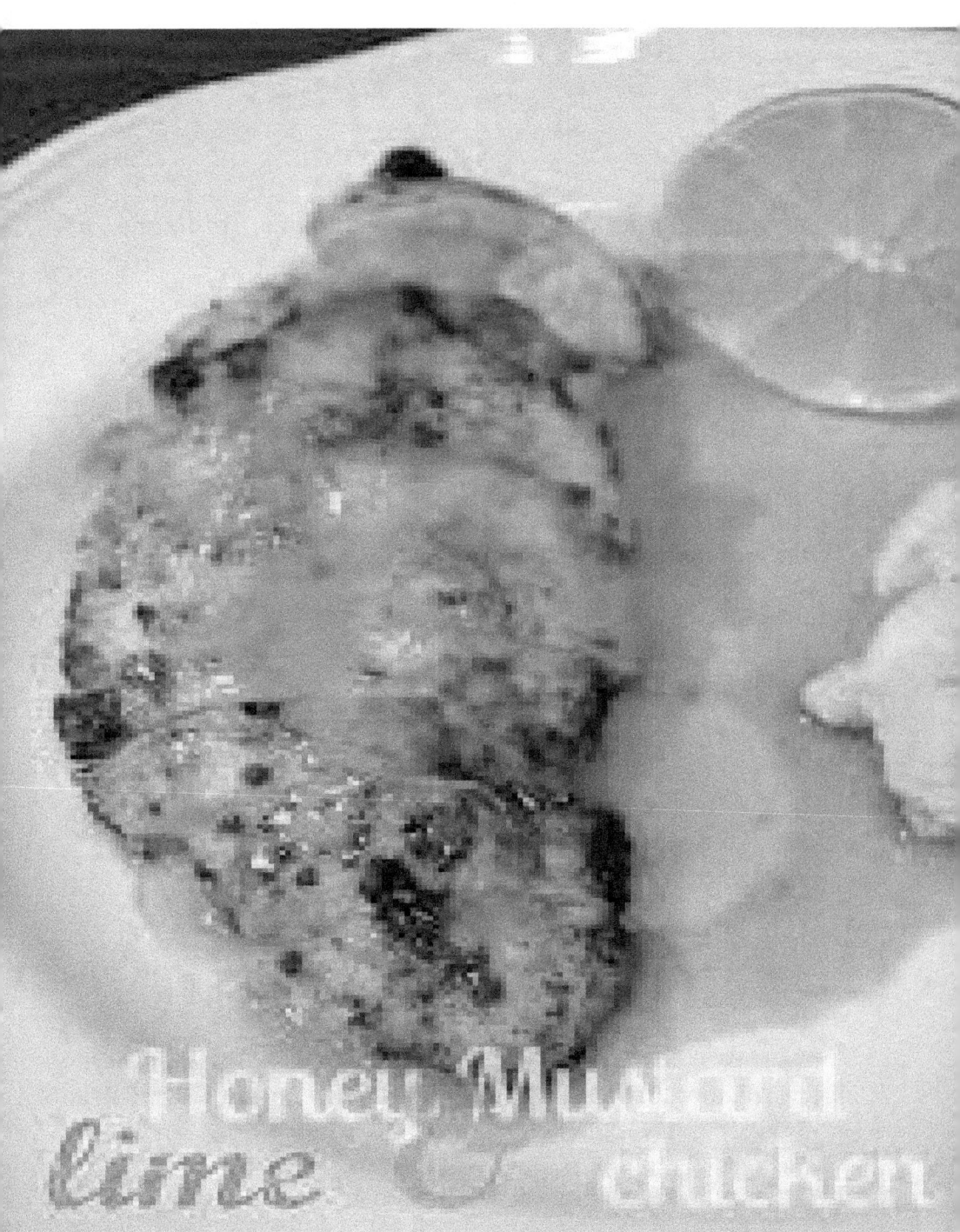

Honey Mustard lime & chicken

Mustard Lime Chicken

Serves 4

Prep time: 20 minutes, Cook time: 30 minutes, Total time: 50 minutes

Nutritional Information Per Serving: *Calories: 200, Proteins: 31g, Carbohydrates: 12 g, Fats: 2.5g*

Ingredients

½ teaspoon of ground black pepper

½ teaspoon of Celtic sea salt

1 tablespoon of chili powder

1 tablespoon of olive oil

¼ cup of Dijon mustard

½ cup of fresh chopped cilantro

½ cup of fresh lime juice

1 pound of skinless boneless chicken breast

Directions

Place salt, pepper, chili, olive oil, mustard, cilantro and lime juice in a food processor. Blend the mixture until everything is well combined.

Use clean water to rinse the chicken breasts. Pat it dry and place it in a 7 x 11 baking dish.

Pour the lime juice marinate over the chicken. Cover the dish and refrigerate it for 15 minutes or up to 6 hours, depending on when you want to prepare the chicken.

Remove from the fridge and bake it at 350 degrees Fahrenheit for approximately 25-30 minutes.

Serve the chicken with cooked sauce spooned over it.

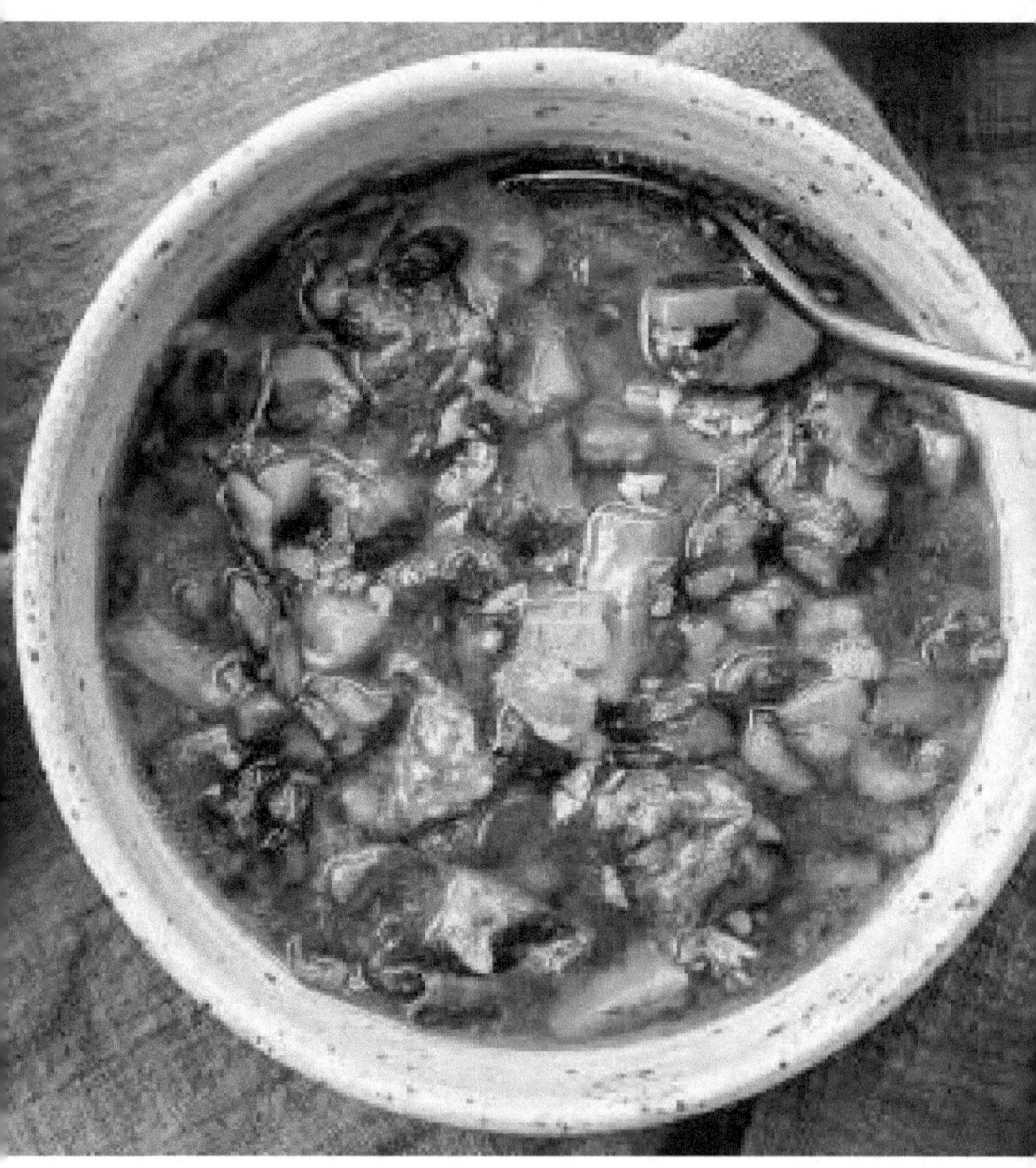

Beef Bourguignon

Serves 6

Prep time: 30 minutes, Cook time: 50minutes, Total time: 1 hr. 20 minutes

Nutritional Information Per Serving: *Calories: 220, Proteins: 27g, Carbohydrates: 6.5g, Fats: 5g*

Ingredients

Salt and pepper

1 teaspoon of dried thyme

1 tablespoon of tomato paste

¾ teaspoon of xanthan gum

¾ cup of dry red wine

3 bay leaves

5 cloves of minced garlic

2 chopped carrots

10 ounces of cremini mushrooms, quartered

1 small onion, chopped

5 strips of diced bacon

1.5-2 pounds of beef chuck roast that is cut into ¾ inch cubes

Directions

Start by seasoning the beef chunks generously with salt and pepper. Set aside.

On a pressure cooker, select the sauté mode for medium heat. Once the display reads HOT, add diced bacon and let it cook until crispy. Stir frequently. This will take you like 5 minutes. Place the bacon on a paper towel-lined plate.

Place the beef on the pot in a single layer and let it cook for a few minutes or until the beef browns. Flip the beef and cook the other side. Once done, place the beef on a plate.

Add garlic and onions. Cook for a couple of minutes or until the onions and garlic soften. Stir frequently. Add tomato paste and red wine. Use a wooden spoon to scrap up the brown pieces stuck at the bottom of the pot. Stir the mixture and check to see if the tomato paste is dissolved. Turn the sauté mode off.

Return the beef back into the pot. Add thyme, carrots and mushrooms and stir everything together. Add bay leaves as topping and then put a lid on the pot. Cook on high pressure for 40 minutes. Follow that with a manual pressure release.

Take the lid off the pot and select the sauté mode. Remove the bay leaves and sprinkle xanthan gum evenly over the pot and stir everything together. Give the stew one minute to boil and thicken as you stir the mixture. Turn the sauté mode off.

Serve the stew into bowls and top them with crispy bacon.

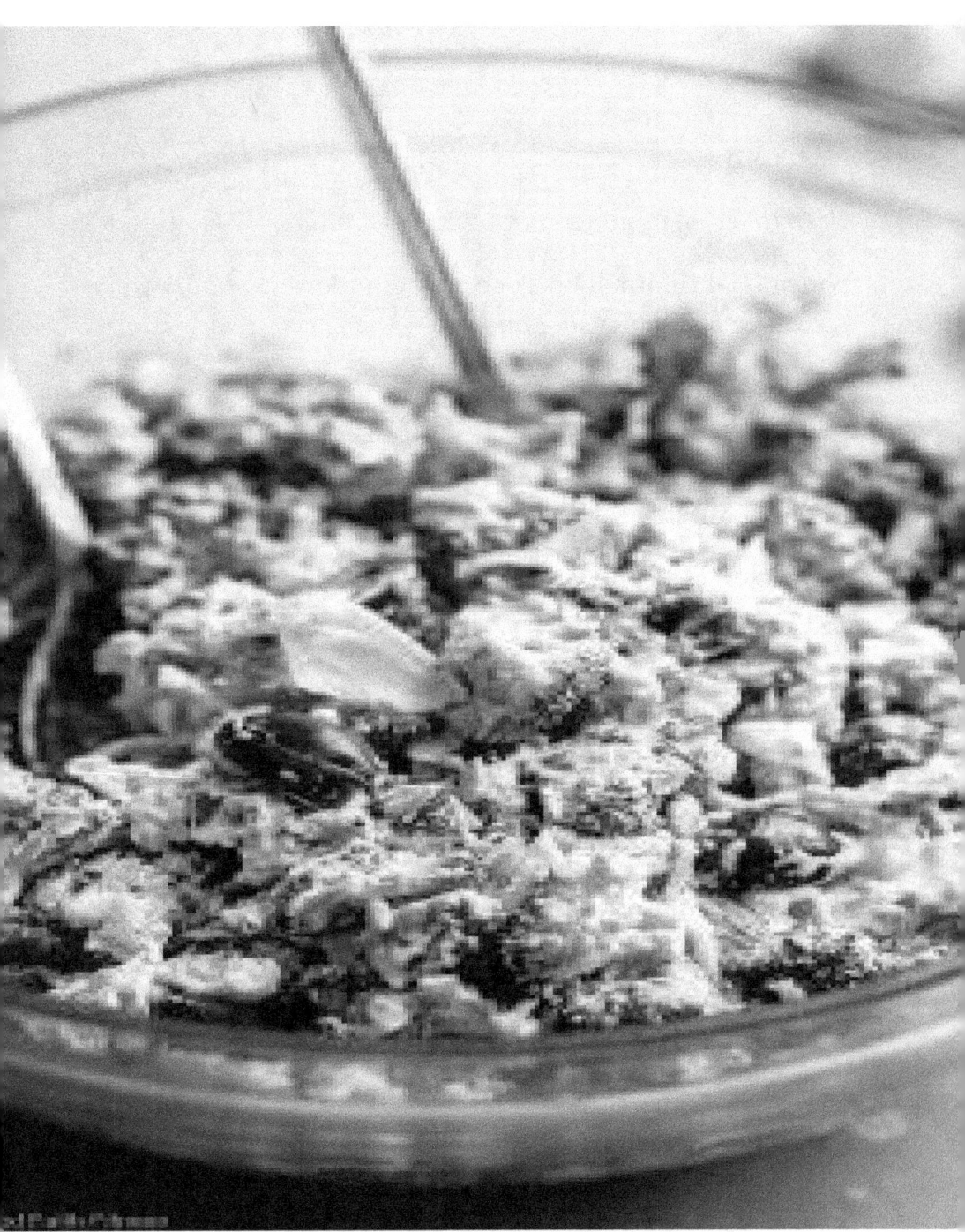

Low Carb Broccoli Salad

Serves 8

Prep time: 25 minutes, Total time: 25 minutes

Nutritional Information Per Serving: *Calories: 290, Proteins: 5g, Carbohydrates: 4g, Fats: 31g*

Ingredients

For the salad

¼ cup of roasted salted sunflower seeds

1/3 cup of diced red onion

½ cup of halved pitted kalamata olives

½ cup of sun-dried tomatoes in olive oil, roughly chopped

½ cup of artichoke hearts marinated in olive oil, sliced

5 cups of broccoli, cut them into small florets

For the dressing

2 tablespoons of oil from the jar of sun-dried tomatoes

Pepper

1 teaspoon of sea salt

1 ½ teaspoons of dried ground thyme

1 ½ teaspoons of dried ground basil

1 ½ teaspoons of fresh garlic, minced

1 ¾ teaspoons of dried oregano

4 ½ teaspoons of Monk fruit

Zest and juice of 1 large lemon

2 cups of plain non-fat Greek yogurt

Directions

Mix together all the salad ingredients in a large sized bowl.

Stir together all the dressing ingredients in a medium sized bowl.

Pour the dressing over the salad. Stir the mixture until everything is well coated.

Cover the bowl and refrigerate for 2 hours or up to overnight. This gives the broccoli time to absorb the dressing and add flavor.

Once ready to eat. Remove the salad from the fridge and serve.

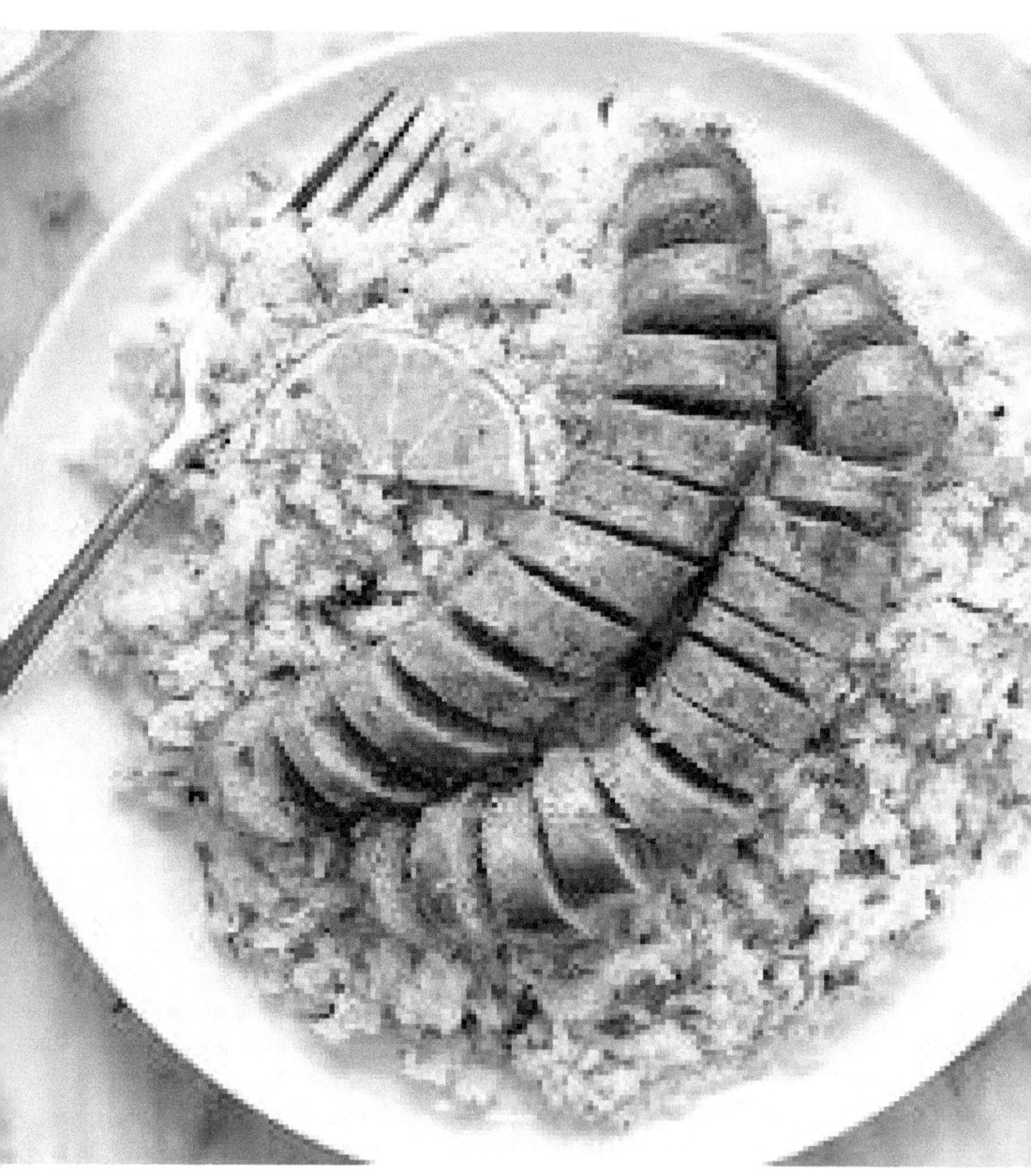

Sausage With Cilantro Lime Cauliflower Rice

Serves 2

Prep time: 5 minutes, Cook time: 20 minutes, Total time: 25 minutes

Nutritional Information Per Serving: *Calories: 60, Proteins: 1g, Carbohydrates: 0.7g, Fats: 4.8g*

Ingredients

Freshly cracked black pepper to taste

1 teaspoon of Italian seasoning

Fresh chopped cilantro

2 tablespoons of fresh lime juice

Zest of ½ lime

1 tablespoon of hot sauce of choice

¼ cup of low sodium chicken stock

3 minced garlic cloves

1 tablespoon of olive oil or butter

½ head of cauliflower, riced

3 or 4 mild Italian sausages

Directions

Place a skillet over medium-low heat. Add ¼ cup of water and bring it to boil. Add the sausages and cover the skillet until the sausages are cooked. Turn the sausages from time to time. Remove the skillet lid and let the water to evaporate. Turn the sausages from one side to another until they are browned. Place the sausages in a plate and set aside.

Use the same skillet to melt olive oil or butter. Add minced garlic and let it cook for 1 minute as you stir occasionally. Add cauliflower rice and toss to coat. Add hot sauce, lime juice, Italian seasoning and chicken broth. Simmer the mixture until the sauce reduces a little bit. This will take you 3-4 minutes.

Add chopped cilantro and lime zest into the cauliflower rice and give the food a quick stir. Season the cauliflower rice mixture with black pepper. Add the sausages into the skillet in order for the sausage to reheat. Heat it for 2 minutes.

Serve the Italian sausage together with cauliflower and cilantro lime. Enjoy.

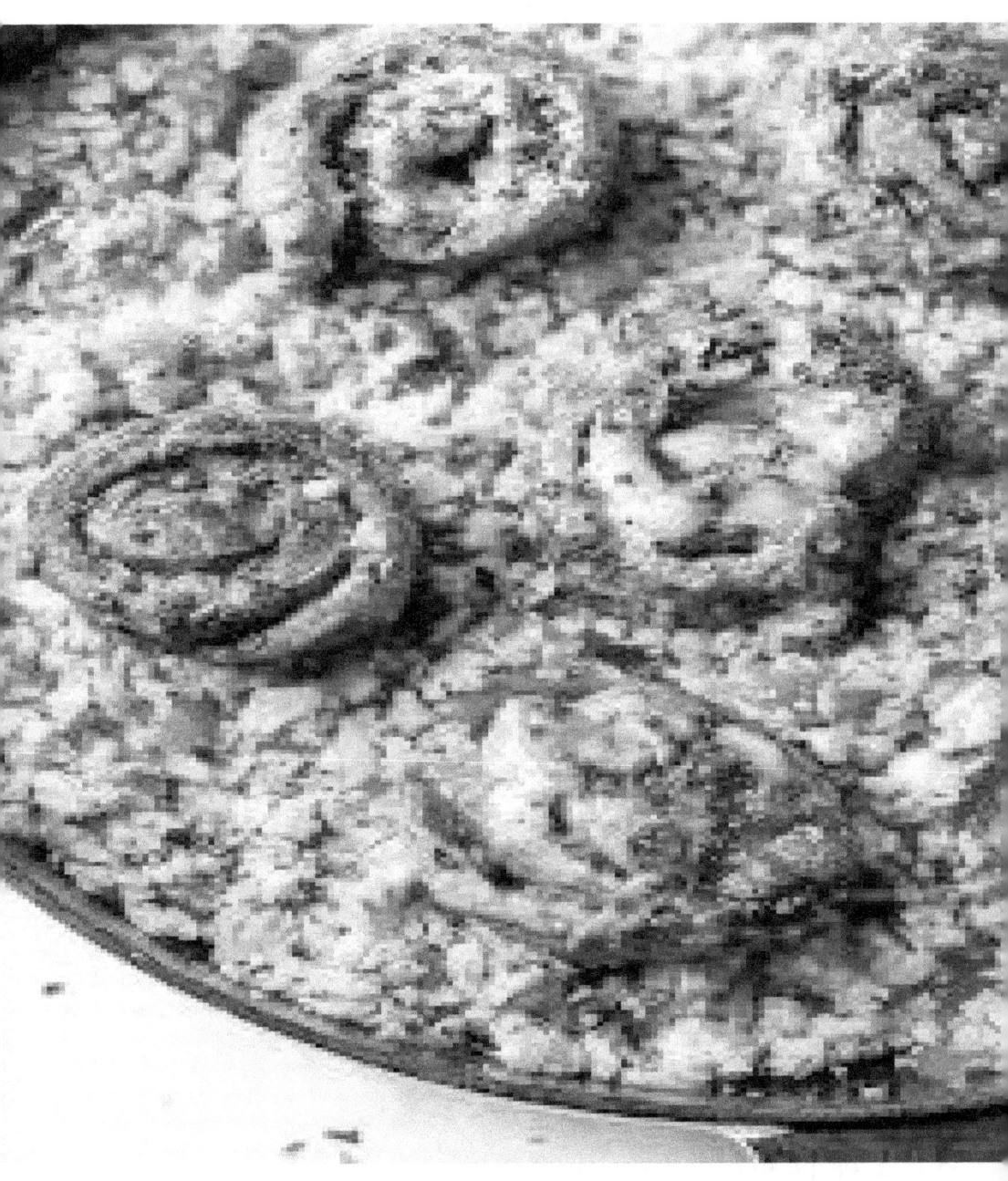

Cauliflower Rice With Cheesy Steak Roll-Ups

Serves 4

Prep time: 15 minutes, Cook time: 15 minutes, Total time: 15 minutes

Nutritional Information Per Serving: *Calories: 416, Proteins: 17g, Carbohydrates: 21g, Fats: 23 g*

Ingredients

The steak rolls

1 cup of shredded mozzarella

½ cup of chopped parsley

3 garlic cloves, minced

1 tablespoon of melted butter

1 lb. of flank steak, sliced lengthwise

The cauliflower rice

Cilantro for garnish

¼ cup of vegetable stock

1 teaspoon of paprika

1 teaspoon of chili powder

1 teaspoon of cumin

½ teaspoon of garlic powder

½ teaspoon of onion powder

½ teaspoon of fine grain sea salt

1 jalapeno pepper, seeds removed and minced

1 red bell pepper, diced

1 small yellow onion, minced

2 tablespoons of olive oil

1 head cauliflower, riced

Directions

Start by combining salt, pepper, oregano, garlic powder, cumin, cayenne, paprika and chili powder in a small bowl.

Use another small bowl to mix melted butter with salt, pepper, parsley and minced garlic.

Place the flank steak on a cutting board. It should be laying down flat with the grain running up and down. Use a cooking brush to brush the steak with the garlic mixture. Place a layer of cheese on top of the steak and tightly roll up the meat. Make sure you cut against the grain when you slice the meat. To help the roll to hold its shape, stick toothpicks on the sides of the roll. Cut in between the toothpicks using a sharp knife.

Place a skillet over high heat. Add the steak rolls and let them sear for about 3 minutes on each side or until a nice crust has developed. Remove the rolls and set aside.

Add 2 tablespoons of olive oil to the same skillet. Add jalapeno, bell pepper, garlic and onion and sauté them until soft. This should take 3 minutes.

Add the cauliflower rice and stir the mixture until the rice is well coated. Cook for 2 minutes as you stir regularly. Add spice mix and ½ cup of vegetable stock. Cook for a few minutes to reduce the juice. Taste and adjust seasoning.

Add the steak rolls to the cauliflower rice and reheat for a few minutes. Garnish the food with parmesan shavings and chopped parsley.

Serve and enjoy.

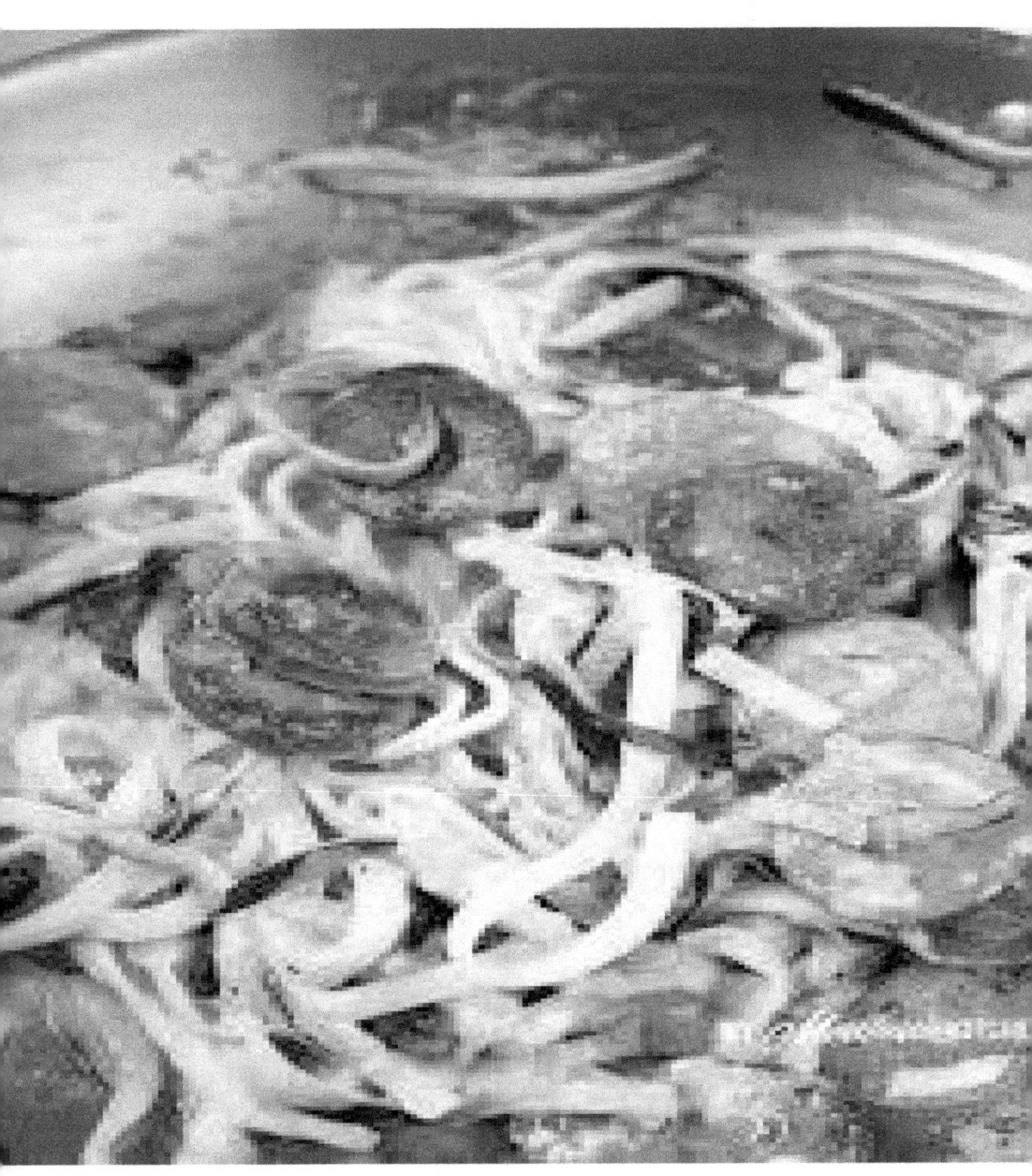

Zucchini Noodles With Sausage Alfredo

Serves 4

Prep time: 15 minutes, Cook time: 20 minutes, Total time: 35 minutes

Nutritional Information Per Serving: *Calories: 583, Proteins: 16g, Carbohydrates: 6.1g, Fats: 52g*

Ingredients

2 medium zucchini spiralized

Salt and pepper

½ cup of freshly grated parmesan

1 cup of heavy whipping cream

3 cloves of minced garlic

2 tablespoons of butter

12 ounce of bulk hot Italian sausage

Directions

Prepare the sausage. Add the sausage in a large skillet over medium heat. Let it brown for 5-8 minutes or until cooked through. Put the sausage on a bowl and leave its grease on the pan.

Add butter in the skillet and let it melt. Add garlic and sauté for 1 minute or until fragrant. Add cream and bring the mixture to a simmer. Reduce the heat to low. Cook for a further 5 or 8 minutes as you whisk the food frequently.

Whisk the parmesan in and season with salt and pepper to taste.

Add the sausage and whisk to combine. If the sauce is too thick, you can add extra cream.

Prepare the zucchini noodles. Use a microwave safe bowl to microwave zucchini noodles on high heat for 2 minutes or until the noodles become tender. Divide the noodles among 4 plates and top each plate with sausage Alfredo. Enjoy.

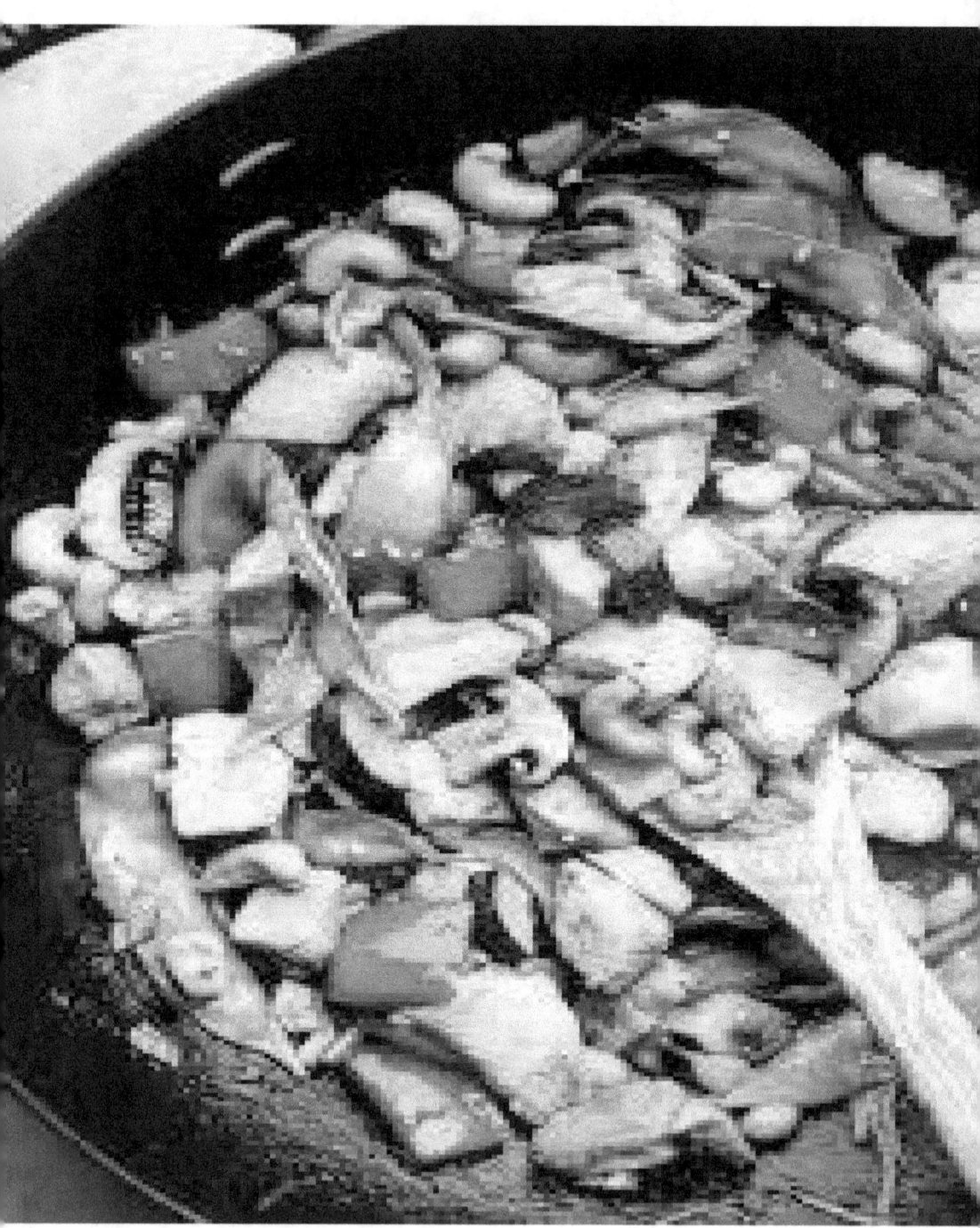

Cashew Chicken Fry

Serves 4

Prep time: 10 minutes, Cook time: 10 minutes, Total time: 20 minutes

Nutritional Information Per Serving: *Calories: 250, Proteins: 28g, Carbohydrates: 2g, Fats: 10g*

Ingredients

Green onions sliced for garnish

2 tablespoons of water

1 tablespoon of cornstarch

1 teaspoon of sesame oil

1 tablespoon of brown sugar

3 cloves of minced garlic

¼ cup of low sodium soy sauce

¾ cup of chicken broth

1 cup of whole cashews

1 cup of snow peas

½ cup of shredded carrots

1 cup of sliced mushrooms

1 red bell pepper cut into one inch cubes

1 zucchini diced

1 pound of boneless skinless chicken breasts that's cut into one inch cubes

1 tablespoon of olive oil

Directions

Start by adding olive oil and chicken in a medium-sized skillet over medium high heat.

Brown the chicken until it's almost cooked through. Add in snow peas, carrots, mushrooms, bell pepper and zucchini.

Cook the food until the chicken is no longer pink and the vegetables are tender.

Add cashews followed by chicken broth, sesame oil, brown sugar, garlic and soy sauce.

Make slurry. Whisk water together with cornstarch in a small bowl.

Pour the slurry in the skillet and stir the mixture until well incorporated. Let the mixture simmer for 2 minutes. The sauce should be thick by then.

Garnish the chicken fry with green onions and serve it over rice.

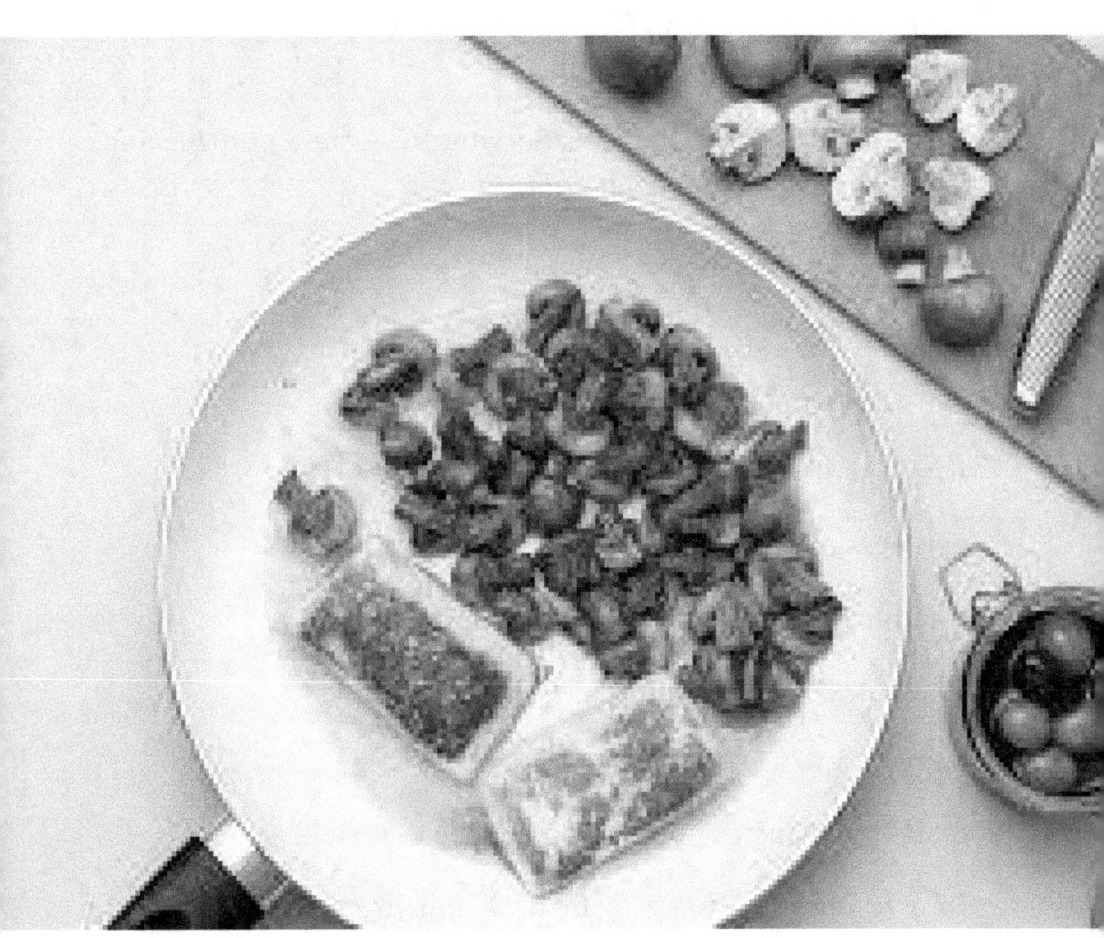

Halloumi Cheese With Mushrooms

Serves 2

Prep time: 2 minutes, Cook time: 10 minutes, Total time: 12 minutes

Nutritional Information Per Serving: *Calories: 591, Proteins: 20g, Carbohydrates: 19g, Fats: 31g*

Ingredients

Optional: ½ cup of mayonnaise

Salt and pepper

10 green olives

3 ounces of butter

10 ounces of halloumi cheese

10 ounces of mushrooms

Directions

Start by rinsing the mushrooms. Slice them.

In a frying pan that can fit both mushrooms and Halloumi cheese, heat a dollop of butter.

Add the mushrooms and fry them for 3-5 minutes or until they turn golden brown. Season the mushroom with some salt and pepper.

Add butter into the frying pan. Let it heat before you add the halloumi. Fry the halloumi for some minutes on each side. As that goes on, stir the mushrooms frequently. Towards the end, lower the heat. Serve with olives and enjoy.

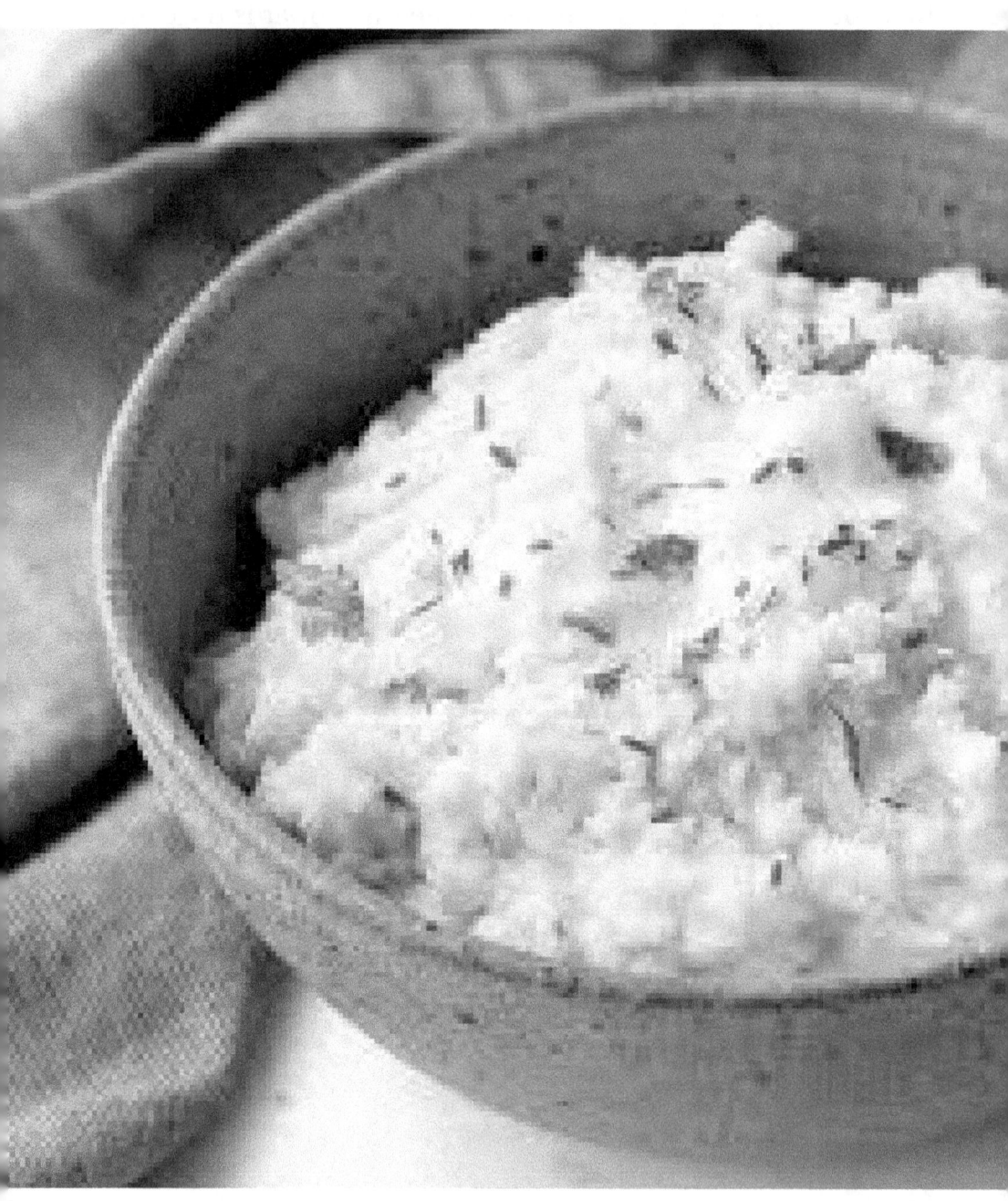

Creamy Cauliflower Mashed Potatoes

Serves 1

Prep time: 10 minutes, Cook time: 15 minutes, Total time: 25 minutes

Nutritional Information Per Serving: _Calories: 107, Proteins: 1g, Carbohydrates: 1g, Fats: 7g_

Ingredients

½ cup of almond milk

1 tablespoon of parmesan cheese

2 tablespoons of grass-fed butter

1 head of cauliflower

Directions

Start by adding broken up pieces of cauliflower into a pot containing water over medium heat and. Bring the water to boil.

As soon as it reaches a boil, bring down the heat and let it simmer for 12-15 minutes or until the cauliflower softens. Drain the cauliflower and transfer it into a large bowl.

Mash the cauliflower to the consistency of your liking using a masher. Add cheese, butter and milk and blend them together. Serve and enjoy.

Alternatively, you can set your oven to broil and place the mashed cauliflower in. Top it with parmesan. Broil on high up to a point where the parmesan starts to crisp.

Keto Snacks & Desserts

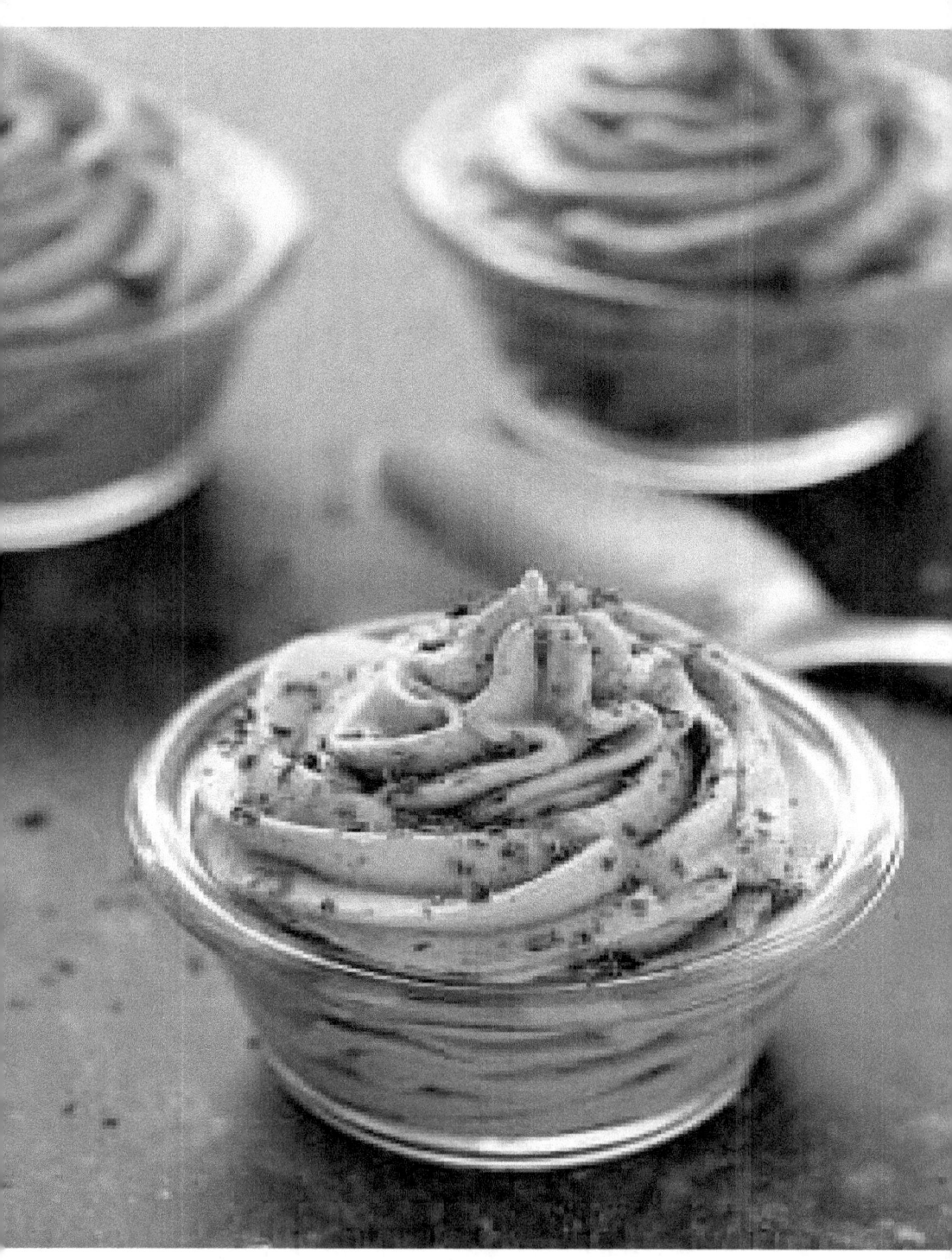

Chocolate Mousse

Serves 8

Prep time: 15 minutes, Total time: 15 minutes

Nutritional Information Per Serving: *Calories: 192, Proteins: 2.4g, Carbohydrates: 4.2g, Fats: 11.1g*

Ingredients

90% of dark chocolate shaved, for garnish

¼ cup of heavy whipping cream

2-3 tablespoons of desired sweetener

1/8 teaspoon of vanilla extract

½ large avocado, pitted

¼ cup of unsweetened cocoa powder

8 ounces of cream cheese block, softened

Directions

Use a handheld mixture to beat together the cream cheese in a medium mixing bowl until it becomes creamy and smooth. As you do that, slowly mix in the cocoa powder. Beat the avocado in and mix until the mixture is creamy smooth. This should take you 5 minutes.

Add some vanilla extract and sweetener and beat the mixture again for 1-2 minutes or until smooth.

Use a separate mixing bowl to whip the heavy cream until it forms stiff peaks.

Transfer the whipped cream into the chocolate mixture and gently fold them together until well incorporated.

Transfer the chocolate mousse into a piping bag and pipe the mousse into desired containers. Garnish with the dark chocolate shavings. Enjoy.

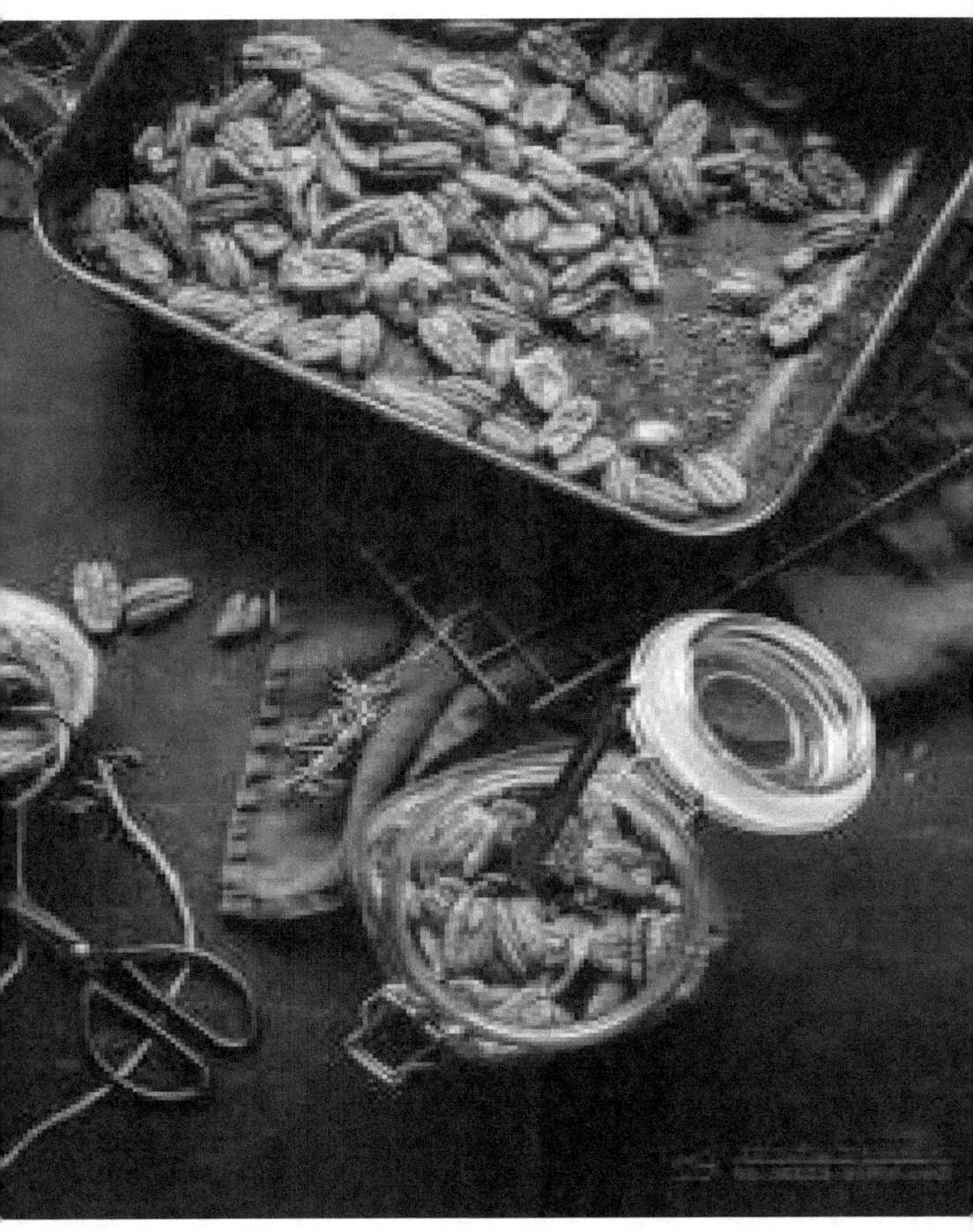

Savory Spiced Pecans

Serves 8

Prep time: 5 minutes, Cook time: 15 minutes, Total time: 20 minutes

Nutritional Information Per Serving: *Calories: 348, Proteins: 4.6g, Carbohydrates: 2.3g, Fats: 36.1g*

Ingredients

Optional: ¼ teaspoon of cayenne pepper

¼ cup of extra virgin oil

2 teaspoon of fresh lemon zest

2 teaspoon of pink Himalayan salt

¼ teaspoon of smoked paprika

¼ teaspoon of onion powder

¼ teaspoon of garlic powder

4 tablespoon of roughly chopped fresh rosemary

4 cups of pecans

Directions

Start by preheating your oven to 180 degrees Celsius or 355 degrees Fahrenheit.

Place the nuts in a large bowl. Add in all the spices except the lemon zest. Pour the olive oil in and stir the mixture thoroughly until the nuts are well coated.

Pour the nut mixture onto a lined oven tray and spread it into an even layer. Place on the oven and bake for 10-15 minutes or until they turn golden and toasty. As the nuts bake, you will need to stir them after every 5 minutes for you to get an even browning. Be careful especially for the last 5 minutes because the nuts can burn.

Remove from the oven and give the nuts a few minutes to cool down. Sprinkle some lemon zest over the nuts and stir. Let them cool completely.

Place them in a jar and enjoy whenever you feel like snacking.

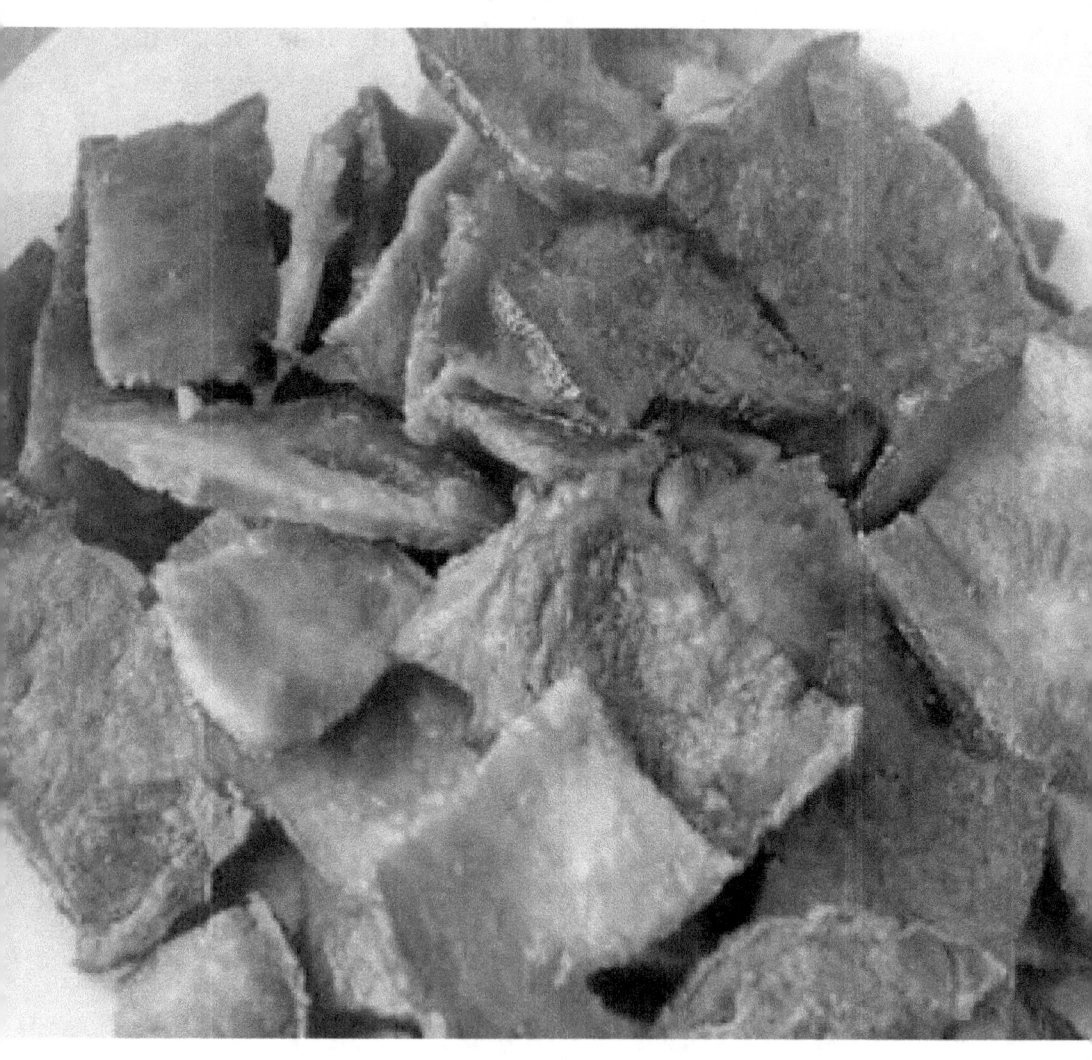

Keto Bacon Chips

Serves 12

Prep time: 5 minutes, Cook time: 10 minutes, Total time: 15 minutes

Nutritional Information Per Serving: *Calories: 110, Proteins: 5g, Carbohydrates: 0g, Fats: 9g*

Ingredients

16 ounces of paleo or whole30 compliant bacon

Directions

Preheat your oven to 375 degrees Fahrenheit.

Use kitchen shears to cut the bacon into one-inch squares.

Line the baking sheet with parchment paper. Lay the bacon chips in one single layer.

Place in an oven and cook until crisp. Serve and enjoy.

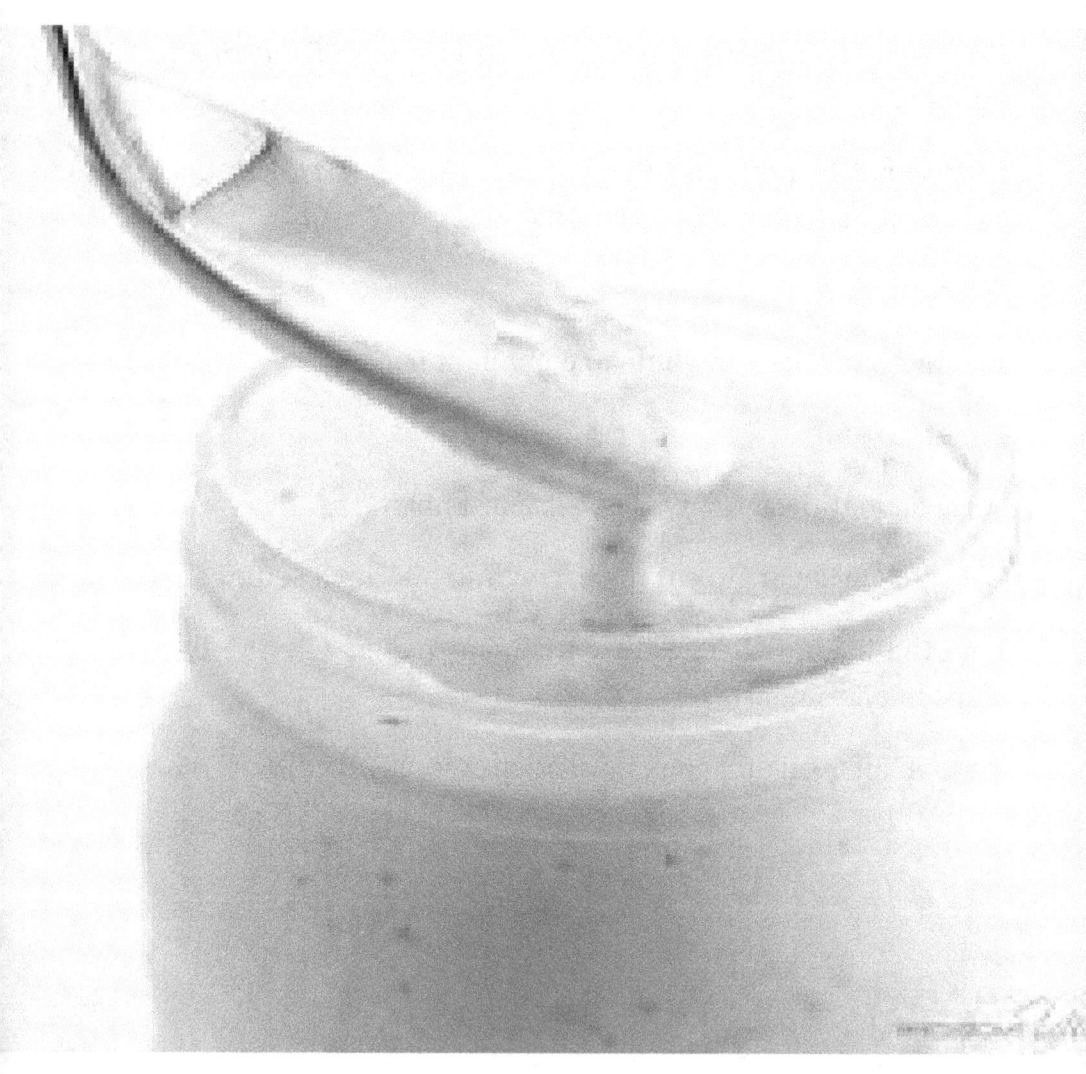

Keto Ranch Dressing

Serves 12

Prep time: 5 minutes, Total time: 5 minutes

Nutritional Information Per Serving: *Calories: 156, Proteins: 0.4 g, Carbohydrates: 0.9g, Fats: 17g*

Ingredients

¼ cup of unsweetened almond milk

¼ teaspoon of black pepper

½ teaspoon of sea salt

½ teaspoon of onion powder

½ teaspoon of garlic powder

1 teaspoon of dried chives

1 teaspoon of dried dill

2 teaspoons of dried parsley

2 teaspoons of lemon juice

½ cup of sour cream

1 cup of mayonnaise

Directions

In a large bowl, whisk all the ingredients together with almond milk being the last one to whisk in. Whisk the almond milk gradually until you reach a consistency that you like.

Put the mixture in the refrigerator and let it cool for 1 hour. This will help the flavors to develop.

Serve as a dip for veggies.

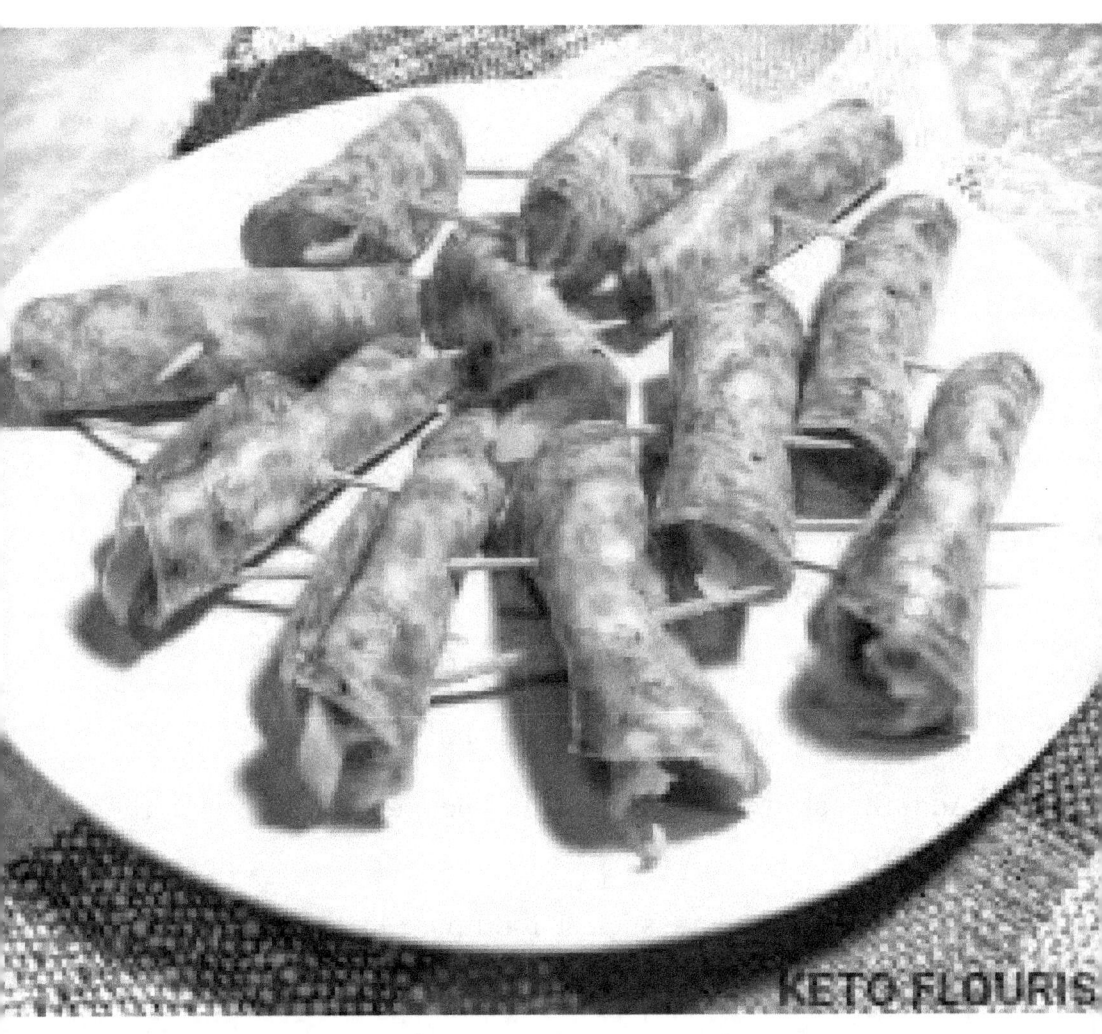

Keto Salami Roll Up

Serves 1

Prep time: 5 minutes, Total time: 5 minutes

Nutritional Information Per Serving: *Calories: 28, Proteins: 1g, Carbohydrates: 0g, Fats: 2.6g*

Ingredients

Peppers for every roll up

½ teaspoon of sliced Pepperoncini

½ teaspoon of cream cheese per roll up

Thinly sliced salami

Directions

Start by laying out your salami on a plate.

Add cream cheese over the salami and spread it out.

Add the slices of pepperoncini peppers and spread them evenly.

Roll the salami and stick a toothpick in the middle of the salami to hold it together. Serve and enjoy.

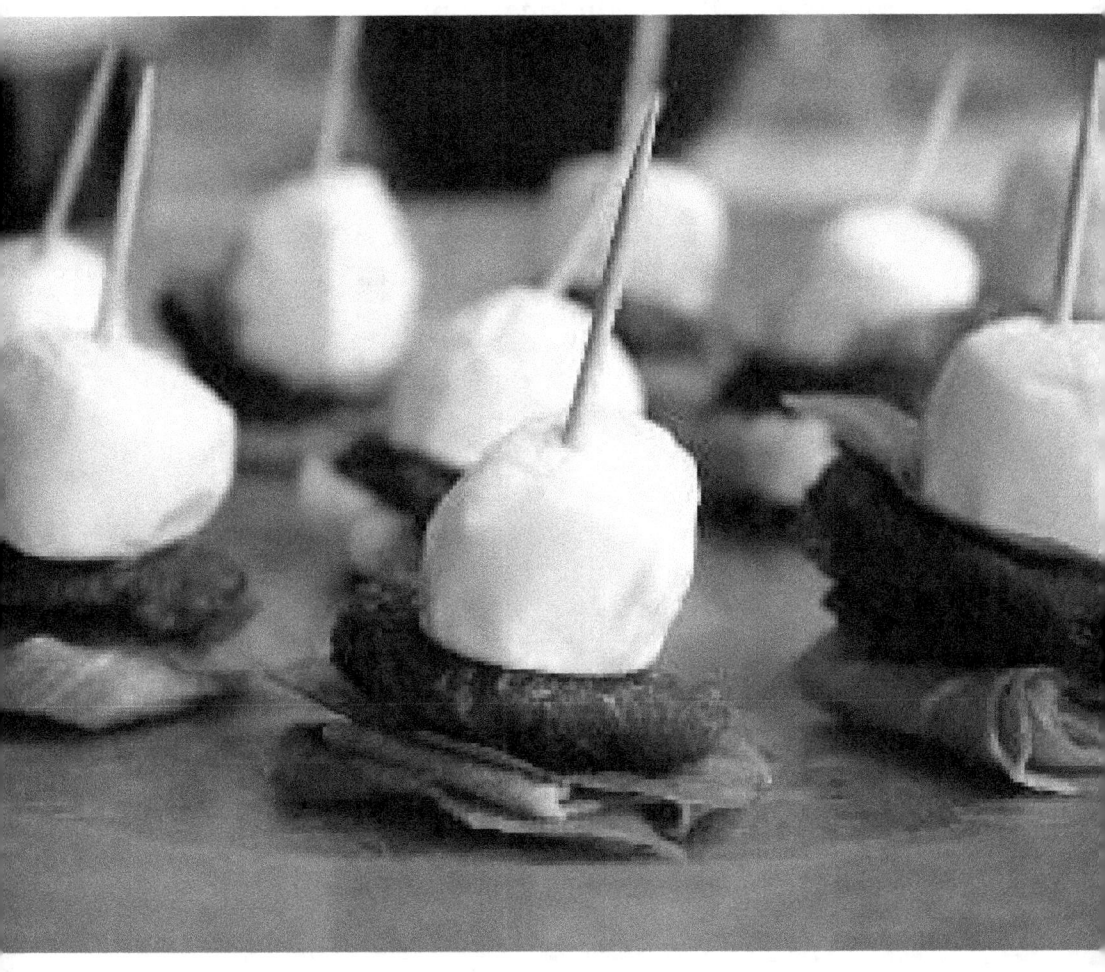

Antipasto Skewers

Serves 1

Prep time: 5 minutes, Total time: 5 minutes

Nutritional Information Per Serving: *Calories: 60, Proteins: 6g, Carbohydrates: 1g, Fats: 4g*

Ingredients

16 basil leaves

16 sun dried tomatoes in oil

16 cillegine (1 inch) mozzarella balls

8 prosciutto slices

Directions

Start by cutting the prosciutto slices in half.

Fold up the prosciutto and lay one sun dried tomato on top of it. Add basil leaf and one mozzarella ball on top.

Skewer with a toothpick and enjoy the snack.

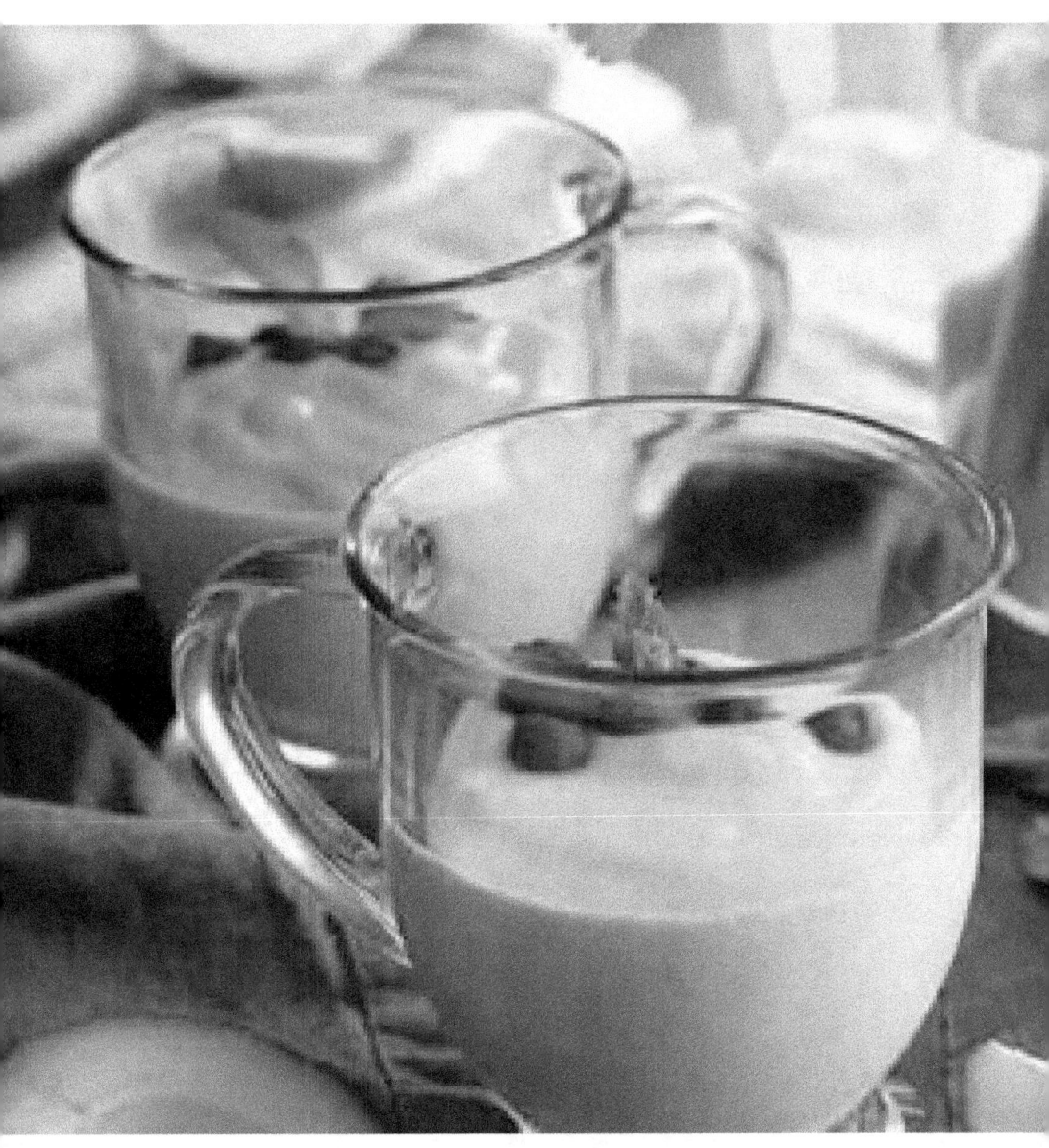

Avocado And Mint Smoothie

Serves 1

Prep time: 2 minutes, Total time: 2 minutes

Nutritional Information Per Serving: *Calories: 223, Proteins: 1g, Carbohydrates: 5g, Fats: 23g*

Ingredients

¼ teaspoon of vanilla

1 squeeze of lime juice

3 springs of cilantro

1-1 1/2 cup of crushed ice

5-6 large mint leaves

Low carb sweetener to taste

½ cup of almond milk

¾ cup of full fat coconut milk

½ of an avocado

Directions

Add all the ingredients in a blender except for the ice.

Pulse on low speed until the mix is completely pureed. Add crushed ice and blend for half a minute. Taste the smoothie and adjust the sweetness.

Serve in a glass and enjoy.

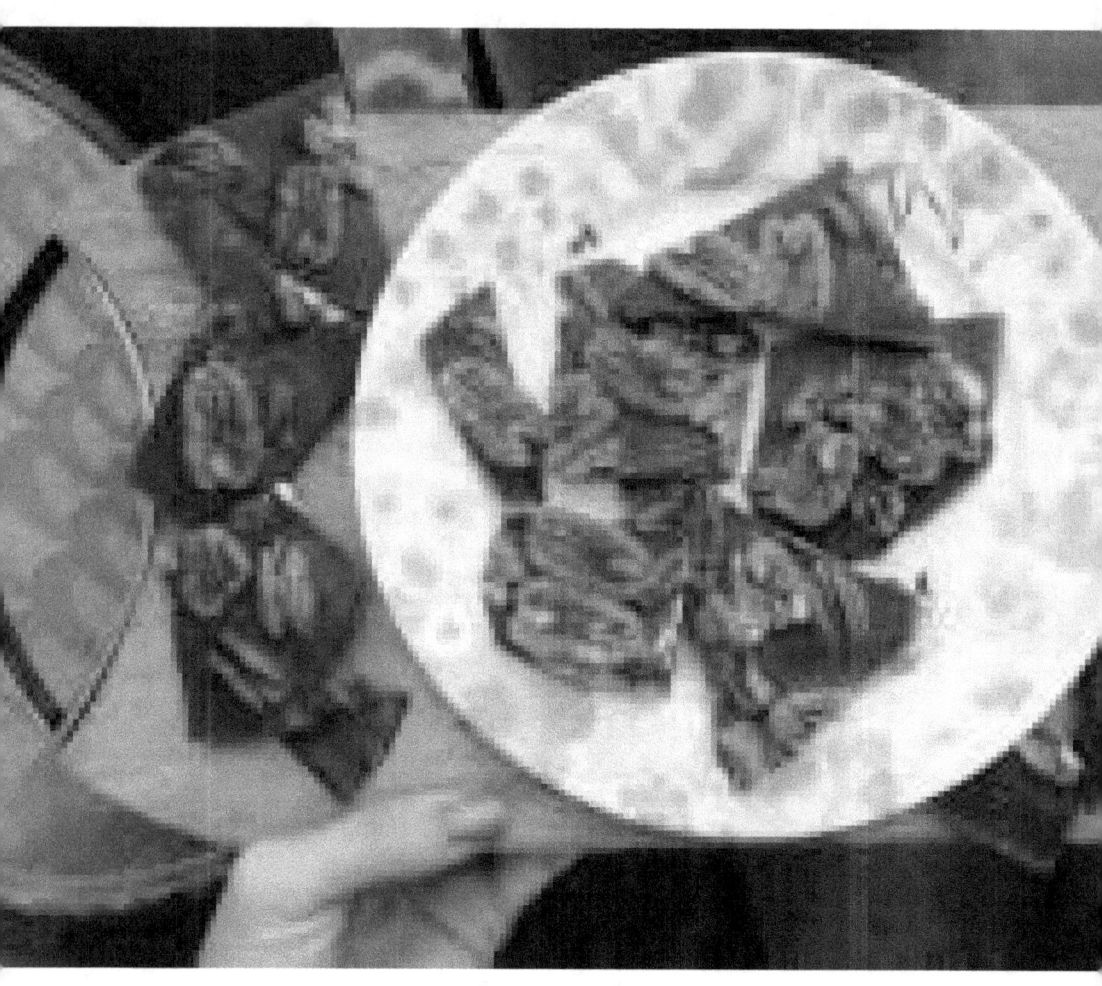

Peanut Butter Pecan Bark (Chocolate)

Serves 25

Prep time: 15 minutes, Cook time: 45 minutes, Total time: 1 hour

Nutritional Information Per Serving: *Calories: 85, Proteins: 2g, Carbohydrates: 1g, Fats: 10g*

Ingredients

½ cup of shredded coconut, unsweetened

1 teaspoon of almond extract

1 teaspoon of vanilla extract

¼ teaspoon of sea salt

½ cup of swerve or stevia

½ cup of creamy peanut butter

¼ cup of unsweetened cocao powder

1 cup of coconut oil

Directions

Start by making the chocolate: Use a skillet placed over medium heat to melt the peanut butter and coconut oil. Stir the mixture until it becomes creamy or until there is no chunk of coconut oil remaining. Add cocoa powder, vanilla extract, almond extract, shredded coconut, stevia and sea salt.

In a lined baking sheet with parchment paper, pour the melted chocolate. Let the chocolate cool and then place it on the fridge to freeze. This should take 45 minutes.

Break the chocolate into pieces and enjoy as dessert. Store the remaining chocolate in a closed container.

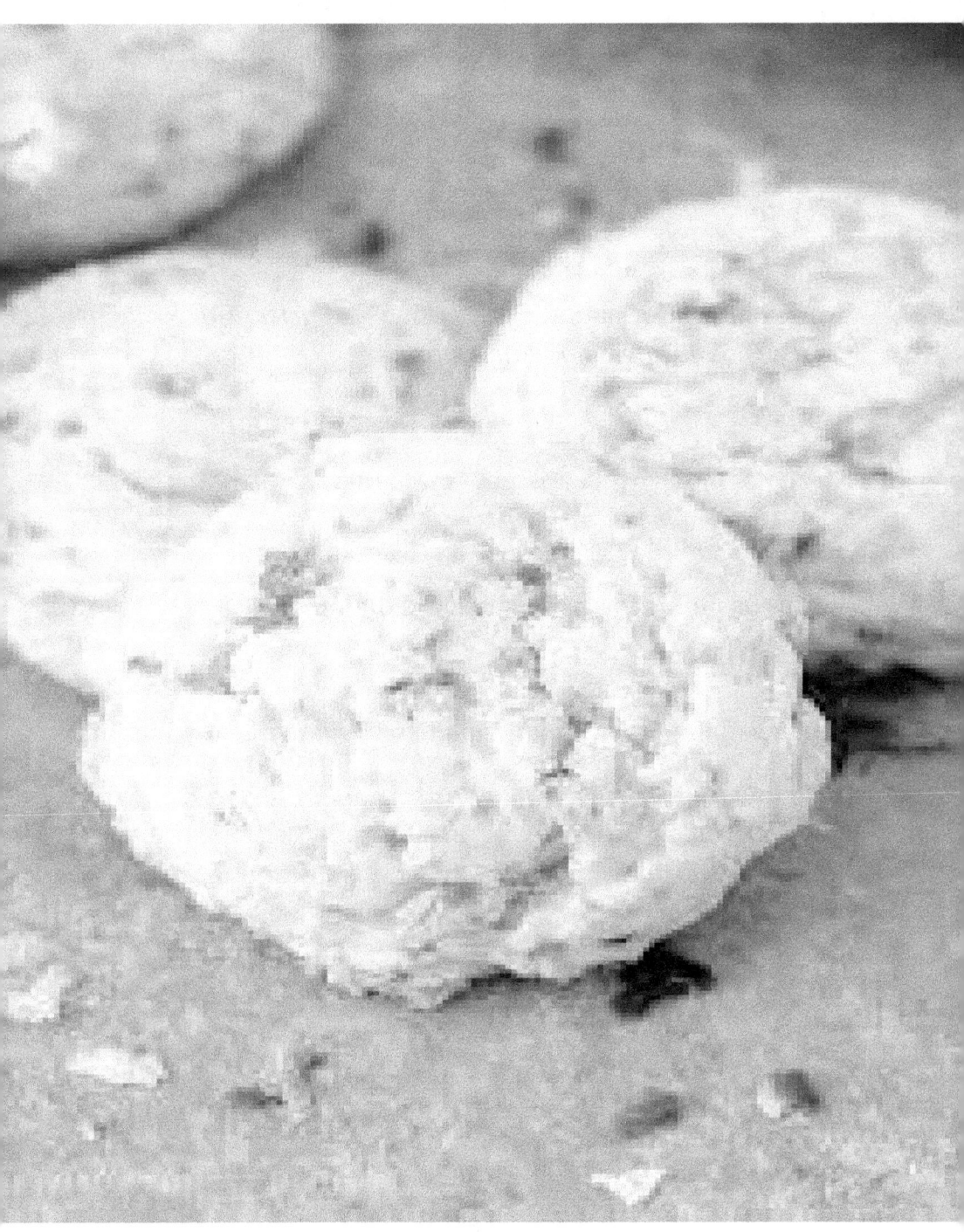

Coconut Cookies

Serving 20 cookies

Prep time: 2 minutes, Cook time: 10 minutes, Total time: 12 minutes

Nutritional Information Per Serving: *Calories: 99, Proteins: 3g, Carbohydrates: 2g, Fats: 10g*

Ingredients

½ cup of monk fruit sweetener maple syrup

1 cup of coconut oil, melted

3 cups of shredded unsweetened coconut flakes

Directions

Line a baking tray or a large plate with parchment paper and set aside.

Combine all the ingredients in a large bowl and mix them together. Wet your hands lightly and start forming small balls with the batter. Place the balls 1-2 inches apart on the lined baking tray.

Use a fork to press the cookies down. Refrigerate the cookies until firm. Serve and enjoy.

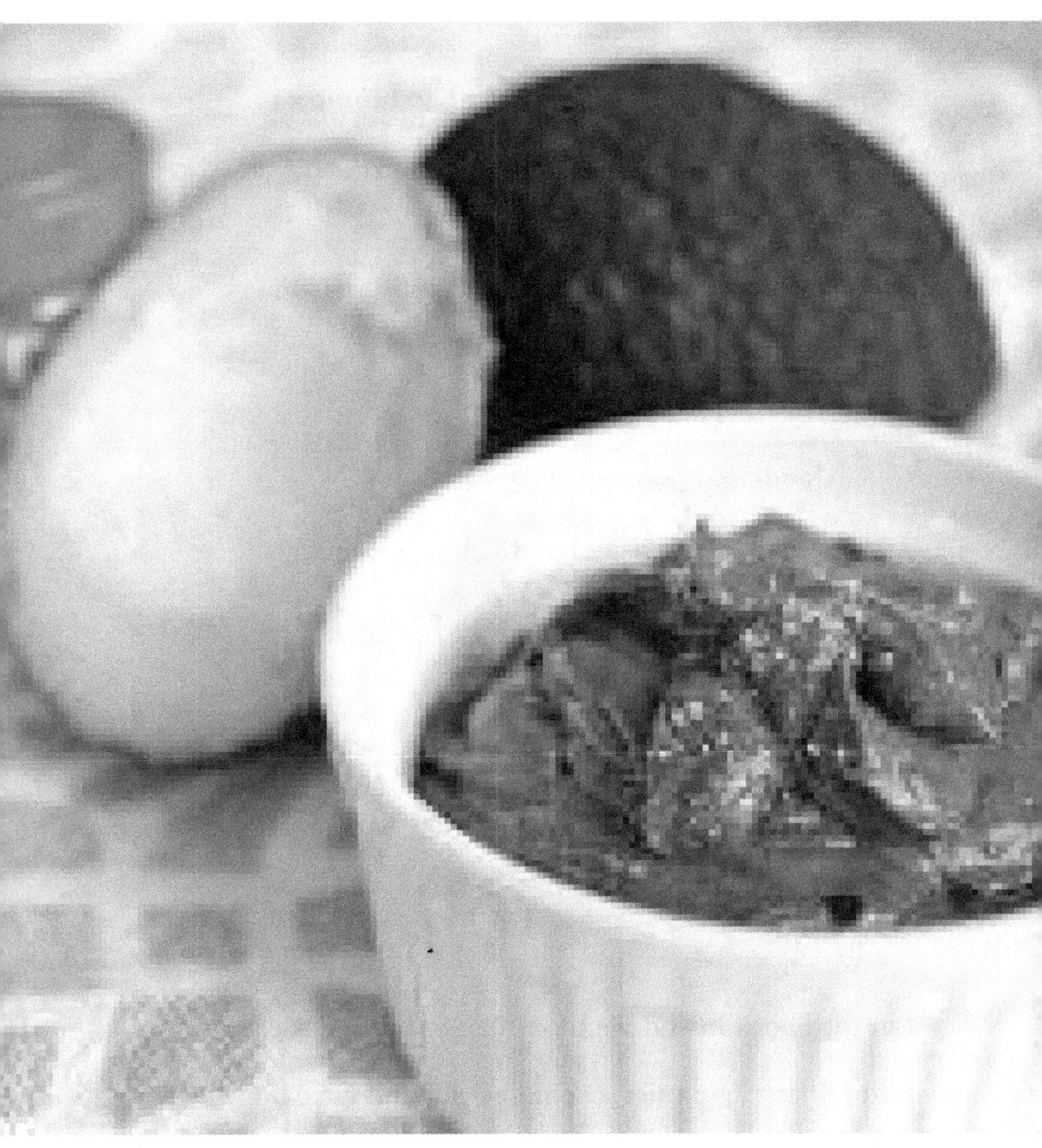

Chocolate Avocado Pudding

Serves 2

Prep time: 10 minutes, Total time: 10 minutes

Nutritional Information Per Serving: _Calories: 160, Proteins: 3g, Carbohydrates: 3g, Fats: 12g_

Ingredients

1 pinch of pink Himalayan sea salt

1 pinch of stevia

½ teaspoon of pure vanilla extract

1 tablespoon of nourished erythritol sweetener

1 tablespoon of unsweetened coconut milk

1 teaspoon of Ceylon cinnamon

1/16 teaspoon of ground cayenne pepper

2 1/2 tablespoon of raw cocoa powder

1 avocado

Directions

Cut the avocado and blend it in a food processor.

Add in vanilla extract, coconut milk and cocoa powder. Blend until smooth.

Add in ground cayenne pepper, stevia, cinnamon and erythritol (or your favorite sweetener). As you blend, keep scraping the sides of the food processor to get the chunks evenly combined.

Serve the avocado pudding with a sprinkle of coarse Himalayan pink sea salt. That will add a flavorful crunch. Enjoy.

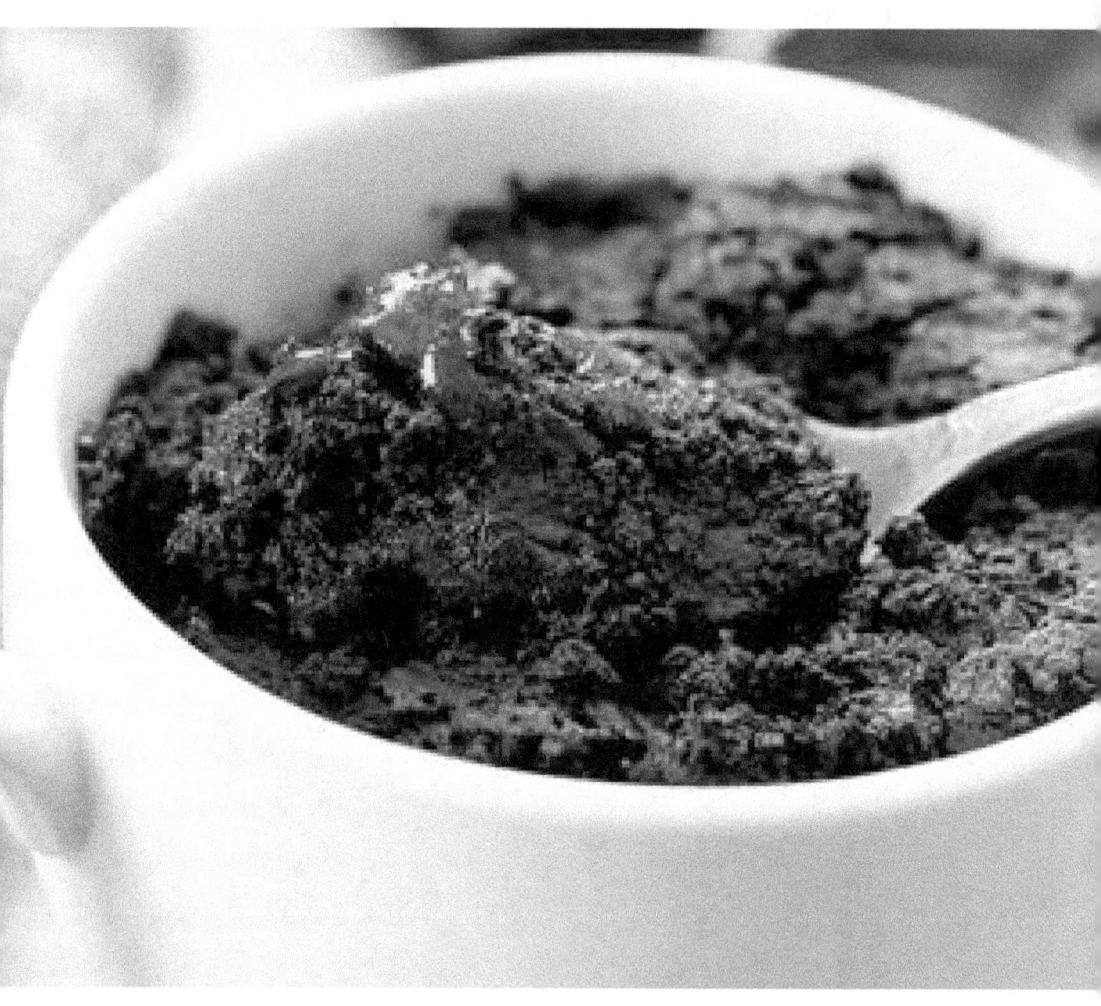

Brownie Mug Cake

Serves 2

Prep time: 1 minutes, Cook time: 1 minutes, Total time: 2 minutes

Nutritional Information Per Serving: *Calories: 101, Proteins: 1g, Carbohydrates: 1g, Fats: 6g*

Ingredients

1 ½ tablespoons of heavy cream

½ teaspoon of baking powder

2 teaspoons of coconut flour

2 tablespoons of unsweetened cocoa powder

½ teaspoon of vanilla extract

1 tablespoon of Sukrin Gold Fiber Syrup

½ teaspoon of coconut oil

Directions

In a medium bowl, add coconut oil and sweetener and place them on the microwave to melt for about 15 seconds.

Stir in vanilla extract. Add in mixed dry ingredients like baking powder, coconut flour and cocoa powder.

Stir in the heavy cream to form a thick brownie batter.

Microwave the mixture for 30-90 seconds or until it reaches a texture that you desire.

Serve while warm. Top with whipped cream if you desire.

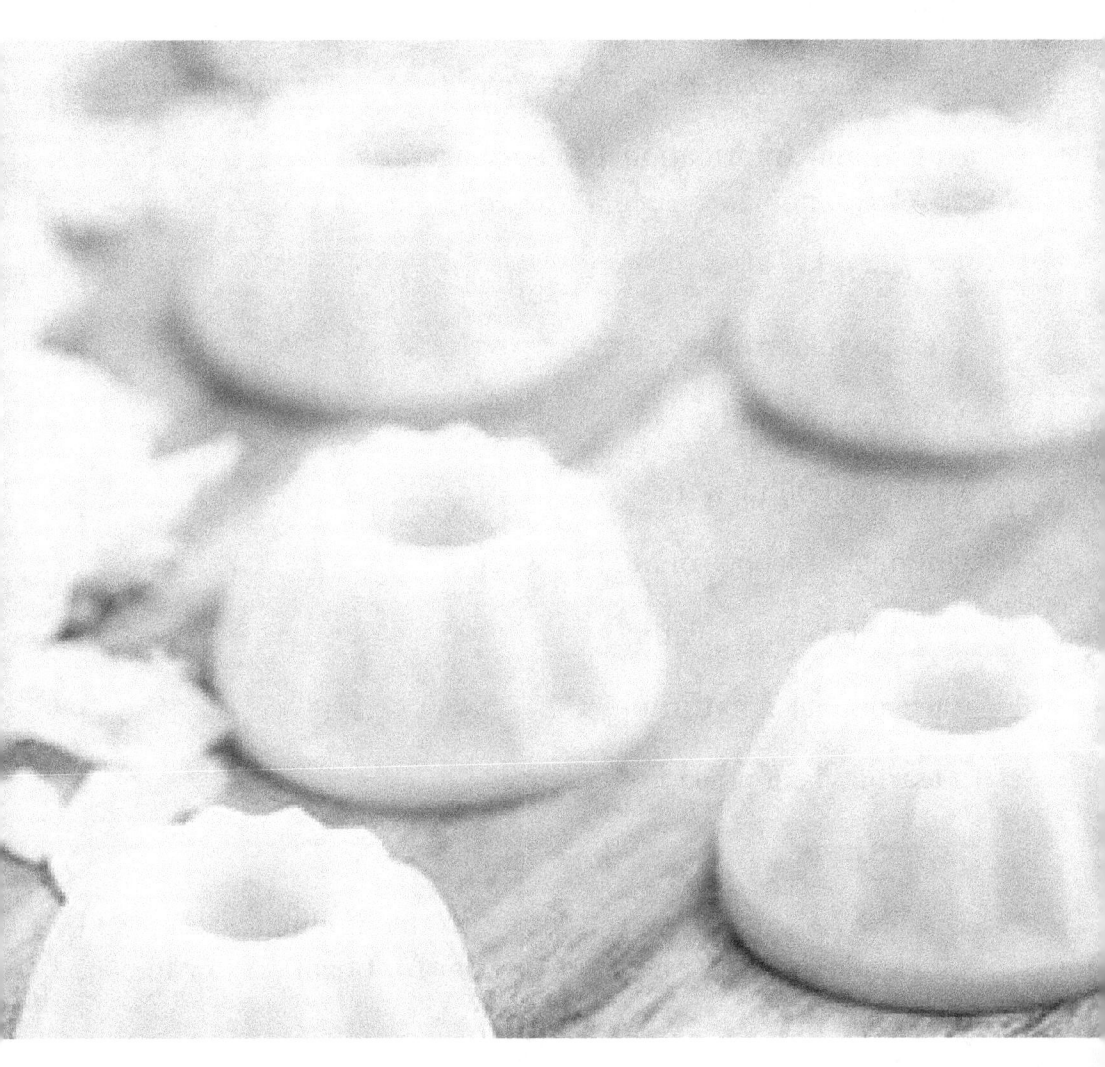

Pina Colada Fat Bombs

Serves 1

Prep time: 1 hour 10 minutes, Total time: 1 hour 10 minutes

Nutritional Information Per Serving: *Calories: 23, Proteins: 2g, Carbohydrates: 0.4g, Fats: 2g*

Ingredients

1 teaspoon of rum extract

½ cup of coconut cream

½ cup of boiling water

Optional: 2 scoops of MCT powder

2 tablespoons of gelatin

3 teaspoons of erythritol

2 teaspoons of pineapple essence

Directions

Dissolve erythritol and gelatin in the boiling water. Add pineapple essence. Add MCT powder (optional). Allow to cool for 5 minutes.

Add rum extract and coconut cream and stir the mix continuously for 2 minutes. Pour the mixture into silicon molds and let sit for 1 hour.

Gently and carefully remove the mold. Enjoy. Store the remaining fat bomb in the fridge.

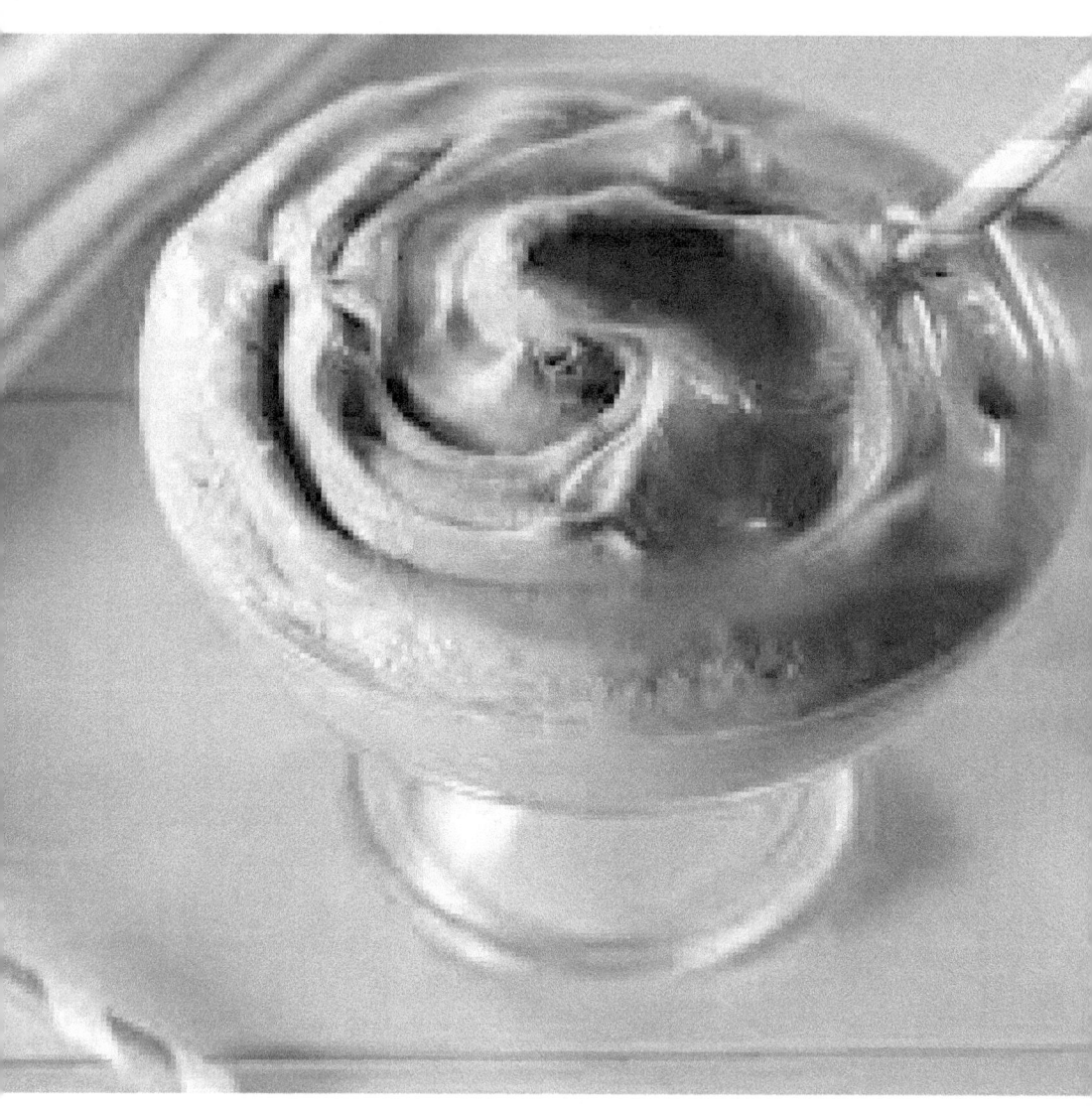

Keto Frosty

Serves 4

Prep time: 10 minutes, Cook time: 35 minutes, Total time: 45 minutes

Nutritional Information Per Serving: *Calories: 103.7, Proteins: 2.1g, Carbohydrates: 2.5g, Fats: 8.6g*

Ingredients

Pinch of kosher salt

1 teaspoon of pure vanilla extract

3 tablespoons of keto friendly sweetener

2 tablespoons of unsweetened cocoa powder

1 ½ cups of heavy whipping cream

Directions

Combine a mixture of salt, vanilla, sweetener, cocoa and cream. Use a whisk attachment or a hand mixer to beat the mixture until stiff peaks form.

Use a spoon to scoop the mixture into a Ziploc bag. Place the bag in the fridge and let it freeze for 30-35 minutes.

Remove from the fridge, snip the tip off from one corner of your Ziploc bag and pipe the mix into a dish. Serve and enjoy.

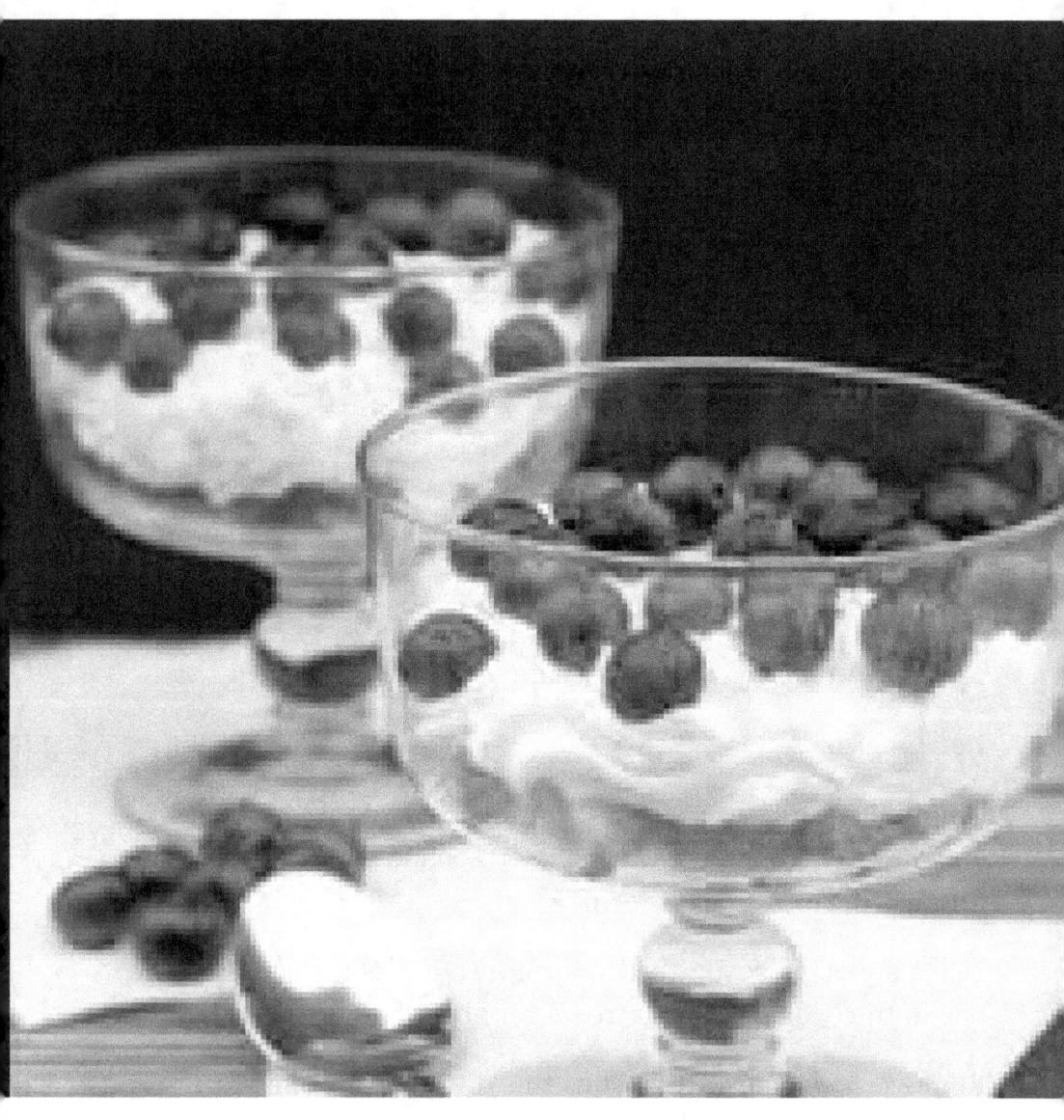

Mascarpone

Serves 12

Prep time: 10 minutes, Total time: 10 minutes

Nutritional Information Per Serving: *Calories: 158, Proteins: 5g, Carbohydrates: 4g, Fats: 15.8g*

Ingredients

1 pint berries (use ½ strawberry and ½ blueberries).

¾ teaspoon of vanilla stevia drops

1 cup of whipping cream

8 ounce of mascarpone cheese

Directions

Use an electric mixer to whip a combination of sweetener, cream and mascarpone in a large mixing bowl.

Pipe into cups and top it with berries. Serve and enjoy.

Motivation

As the old adage goes, 'nothing in life is easy'. That statement fits the keto diet experience like a glove.

Getting into the keto diet has never been easy. This is because it involves you leaving behind a diet that your body was used to and transitioning into a whole new diet that your body is not familiar with. Therefore, it definitely won't be a smooth sail when you first adopt the keto diet.

The question is; how can you deal with the unavoidable challenges that come with transitioning to a keto diet; with the biggest challenge of all being you being able to eat right and keeping your body in the metabolic state of ketosis?

The answer is motivation. As you have heard, going keto can be hard so what you need to get through all the challenges that will come your way is motivation.

Where will you find the motivation? Below are factors that can help you be motivated and stay motivated.

✓ **Joining a social support group**

A social support group is a gathering of like-minded people who come together to talk about things that affect their common interest. In keto, there are different platforms that offer keto support groups. Some of these platforms include Facebook, Instagram and Twitter.

So what you can do is to search for them and join. But why are they important?

As a beginner, a support group is very important to you. This is because it gives you an opportunity to meet people that are experienced in keto dieting. This means you will have people who can answer your questions and guide you through various day to day challenges.

Apart from that, these people also educate you about what is to come. They tell you how they handled different hurdles and even offer you advice on what is the best thing to do in certain situations. That immense support encourages you and motivates you to keep on following the keto diet because people around you have done it and succeeded in it.

✓ Create a positive environment

You may not know this but you can also motivate yourself when on a keto diet. How? Well, you do that by creating a positive and motivational environment for yourself.

For instance, you can stick messages of encouragement in places that you spend the most time of your day in. A good example of these places is your bedroom, your office, on the fridge and in the kitchen. Stick messages like, 'Say no to sugar', 'hard work pays', 'you are what you eat', 'my goal is to lose 10 pounds in the month of October' and 'patience pays'. Those messages help you stay focused and motivated.

✓ Have a weight loss journal

Another way you can self-motivate yourself is by keeping a weight loss journal. This is where you record your progress. This book is nice because it makes you see the fruits of following a keto diet. For instance, imagine you recording that you are 120 pounds and you know that last time you weighed yourself you were 143 pounds. It will feel good right? That is how the weight loss journal encourages you.

✓ Celebrate your success

For you to stick to a keto diet, you must learn to celebrate your success. Otherwise, you may one day look back and wonder what the need for a keto diet is. What you should learn to do is to celebrate the weight you have lost after every month. Choose something that you really want to have and gift yourself that when celebrating. For instance, you can go to watch a movie courtesy of your victory or take yourself to the restaurant and eat your favorite meal. That will definitely encourage you to keep on following the diet.

Those are the four things that you can do to motivate yourself when you start following a keto diet.

As a beginner, there are two things that you must do to be successful in keto dieting.

- You need to **establish why you want to lose weight**. Are you doing it to get into your wedding gown, are you doing it to reduce the chances of developing a weight related health condition or do you just want to impress girls with your body? Asking yourself this question is important because it makes you know why you are following a keto diet and that makes you want to work even harder in order to succeed on the keto diet.

- You need to **have a goal**. Ask yourself what you want to accomplish in a keto diet. Do you want to lose 50 pounds, do you want a masculine body or do you just want a healthy body. A goal helps you stay focused and that's what you need as a newbie in keto diet.

These two factors above are my take-home advice for you; know why you are following a keto diet and know what your goal is.

Conclusion

We have come to the end of the book. Thank you for reading and congratulations for reading until the end.

It is possible for you to lose as much weight as you want on a keto diet. All you need to do is to follow the diet strictly without trying to 'cut corners'. So if you have been struggling with excess weight, you can now courageously say good bye to through following a keto diet.

If you found the book valuable, can you recommend it to others? One way to do that is to post a review on Amazon.

Click here to leave a review for this book on Amazon!

Thank you and good luck!